Heroin, AIDS and Soc

HEROIN, AIDS AND SOCIETY

Roy Robertson

HODDER AND STOUGHTON
LONDON SYDNEY AUCKLAND TORONTO

British Library Cataloguing in Publication Data

Robertson, Roy
  Heroin, AIDS and society.
  1. AIDS (Disease) – Transmission
  2. Heroin habit
  I. Title
  362.2'93   RA644.A25

  ISBN 0 340 39708 X

First published 1987

Photoset by Rowland Phototypesetting Ltd,
Bury St Edmunds, Suffolk.
Printed in Great Britain for
Hodder and Stoughton Educational,
a division of Hodder and Stoughton Ltd,
Mill Road, Dunton Green, Sevenoaks, Kent,
by Richard Clay Ltd, Bungay, Suffolk.

Contents

For my wife Liz and son Jamie

Acknowledgements

This book was written during a busy year in a general practice. Without the support of the following people it would not have been possible. In particular, Aidan Bucknall and Martin Plant provided many of the ideas and much of the encouragement to write them down. Without complaint, the partners of the West Granton Medical Group have supported a project which has continually put them under pressure and the responsibility for patients' welfare has been theirs.

Merrill Whalen, Hilda Purdie and Elaine Smith have done the typing and made sensible suggestions throughout.

The project has been funded since 1984 by the Chief Scientist Office of the Scottish Home and Health Department and more detailed data is available in our various reports to that department. I am very grateful for their support.

Many others have given generously of practical and moral support: Anthony Thorley, John Strang, Tom McGlew, John Howie, George Bath, Heather Black, Beverley Davitt and Neil Stewart. Any faults in the book are entirely my own responsibility.

Introduction

During the post war decades the awareness of a drug abuse problem has been constantly present in many societies. It has waxed and waned in importance and continually changed in nature, but steadfastly refuses to go away despite much effort by agencies of all types. Solutions have been proposed and methods implemented to control or to manage those indulging in such damaging behaviour. Some of these have been effective, some little short of disastrous and some have changed our conception of the problem either by shedding new light or by providing information which changed our views.

At no other time has there been so much confusion about drug abuse. From being a clear cut problem of too many tablets being sold to too many people, with an obvious solution of restricting supply, we are now in an era where even the notion of a drug has to be analysed before we can determine whether or not it is a problem. Should we be concerned about cannabis or cocaine or is heroin the real danger? Many more deaths are caused by cigarettes and alcohol, so are these the real issues? Perhaps there is a conspiracy to cover up the damaging effects of drugs or perhaps it is just our cloudy vision.

It is not the intention of this book to present the story of use and abuse except when that relates to how and why drugs are used. It is not meant to be an academic account of facts and figures relating to deaths and disasters of heroin abuse; these are graphically and lucidly accounted for elsewhere. Rather, it is hoped to present a series of discussions, under certain topical headings, in order that debate can be stimulated as to why the professionals and the public behave as they do. Also, it is hoped that it will draw attention to the difficult and confusing areas that prevent clear understanding and therefore definitive action in the various areas of discussion.

As society evolves, concepts and values change and mature. The sudden onset of heroin use in most parts of the Western world has presented a large, alarming and demanding set of social, medical and political problems. To take all these on board at once is difficult, if not impossible, for any community and cannot be done without information and discussion. It is this discussion which we hope to stimulate, even if only in a small way. The problems, however, change constantly and attitudes and responses must do the same.

The dangers of neglecting the problems posed by drugs such as heroin are great and the consequences of making the wrong policy decisions and pursuing an incorrect line of approach are constantly in the minds of those in political control. The price of failure is high, both in terms of society and the future of any political career. Much use has been made of law and order as a vote-winner and this is nowhere more evident than with the current administrations in European and American countries. Hindsight, however, demonstrates that mistakes have been made and this is manifest in many of the leading Western capital cities. Of greater concern is the growing belief that the same mistakes are still being made, but on a bigger scale and with more damaging implications for the future.

What will emerge in the last years of the twentieth century in the field of heroin use can only be guessed at but, for many reasons, attitudes will change and fear and prejudice may be replaced by understanding and concern. The stage is set in all sections of society for a new approach towards the substances which are used or abused, and this will start when perspectives are altered by a clear understanding of the facts about the dangers, the causes and the outcomes for those involved.

This book is based on the experience gained in a Scottish general practice not previously involved with drug takers other than those on drugs prescribed by the Health Service. The explosion of the availability of heroin in the early 1980s has thrown a new group of professionals and volunteers into this problem. In general practice, information is systematically gathered on an individual and family basis over many years. This allowed for a detailed research study, including many previously obscured facets, of those using drugs like heroin. In addition, because of the position of general practice, immediate assembling of the facts given in the text was possible. These data therefore apply to the beginning of an epidemic of heroin use and follow its course as time goes on.

The heroin problem in many Western countries has actually been a series of minor epidemics, occurring and overlapping geographically and temporally. Much research has studied the effects of heroin on individuals after the epidemic phase has passed and often when they have been using heroin for many years. This study observes the individuals from the start of their drug taking and therefore has a unique perspective.

To fill in many areas of confusion about why a discrete group of youngsters in a provincial centre should start using heroin has been the main interest. The problems encountered as time goes by have been tabulated and in many cases, such as those tragic deaths in young drug takers, the final outcome is already apparent.

The outcome for the survivors is now of importance as many have become infected with the virus responsible for AIDS. Sometime in 1983, when many of these people were just beginning to inject heroin, this virus was introduced into the community. Needle and syringe sharing was common at the time and lack of knowledge regarding the dangers of this practice facilitated the rapid spread of the infection.

The events of the next few years therefore will not represent a pattern demonstrated in other epidemics of heroin use. Some will survive and many have already escaped uninfected and apparently resolved to avoid heroin for ever. A large group however are infected with the AIDS virus and many continue to use drugs by injection.

There is now a new factor with, at the present time, more unknowns than answers. With a unique starting point because of its situation, this research will continue to a unique conclusion over a period of perhaps many years.

1 The Nature of Drug Dependence

Faced with a situation new to our personal experience we all react by attempting to fit it into our existing understanding of the world. We may initially analyse it in gross terms and our immediate response may be revulsion, disgust, interest or acceptance, depending upon our orientation to the situation or our previous experience and knowledge. Further, more detailed information may alter or modify our initial assessment. In the light of important new data, we might choose to completely change our viewpoint or to reject the contradictory evidence in favour of our first assessment. Often, information which represents a threat, real or imagined, to the stability of our lives will be rejected, not because it is untrue but because of the discomfort and anxiety which it engenders.

People therefore are reluctant to change and to accept new points of view or new situations and society, being made up of individuals, will move in a new direction only when the considerable force of many individuals is exerted. This is a necessary part of the structure and functioning of socialized humanity.

Change, however, does occur but depends very much on the information available to people, whether they are in a position to make or influence policy, or are part of a tide of public opinion. Sources of information are therefore a critical part of the workings of civilization and the recognition of this is apparent in the continual quest for knowledge in all spheres of human life.

However, in some areas, and the world of heroin use is one of these, there exists a counterforce designed specifically to prevent or distort information available to society. It is very much in the interests of the underground organizations to perpetuate confusion and lack of understanding in the minds of the public and in those of drug users themselves. Additionally, the illegal nature of heroin and heroin use provides further obstacles in the gathering of accurate, relevant or interesting data. Certain areas become available for study and therefore form a basis for understanding but other larger parts of the jigsaw remain obscure and prevent a clear view of the picture. Slowly one might expect the pieces to fit together and reveal the whole but this depends upon gathering different pieces of the jigsaw rather than the same ones again and again. Research can only analyse the data available to it, and in the field of heroin use this has tended to be that presenting to medical or psychiatric, prison or social services.

Much, therefore, is known about heroin users when they are in crisis. Much is known about how they behave in prison or in hospital. More recently, attempts to understand behaviour leading to heroin use have demonstrated much about causative factors. Large areas, however, remain cloudy to our vision of the heroin phenomenon. Perhaps the information is there and, for the reasons discussed above, we are unwilling to see it, or perhaps real knowledge is eluding us.

Available Information

Extensive research and observation over the past 20–30 years have given us much understanding of heroin users and the nature of the drugtaking underworld. Stimson's study of London heroin users over a ten year period (1969–1979) forms the basis of the picture which has emerged of a 'typical' heroin user:

> 'The typical addict patient was male, twenty five years old, born in this country, single, likely to have been separated from one or both parents and left secondary modern school at fifteen. He started using drugs at sixteen, heroin at nineteen, and had used heroin for about five years. Before he started using heroin he had been convicted of an offence not connected with drugs. He was unemployed or only casually employed, and supported himself from a variety of sources including crime.
>
> In addition to heroin he received methadone on prescription, however he did not confine his drugs to those being prescribed for him. He had a good deal of contact with other addicts, injected in their company, and did not inject in a sterile manner. He attempted abstinence but had chronically relapsed, and was often in hospital for treatment of conditions associated with drug use.'

Other studies in Europe and America have substantiated much of this information. They all would admit, however, that this stereotype addict is not necessarily the only heroin user and, furthermore, that the group studied are, in general, those who experience problems with heroin use and therefore present themselves to doctors, police or social services. An obsession with the stereotype has often caused us to overlook the other, often substantial, group of heroin users who do not necessarily comply with that pattern. Although it has been stated many times in many eminent research publications that these non-dependent individuals exist, the concentration of society has been repeatedly drawn to the chaotic, destructive and damaging section of heroin takers and the evidence pointing to the persistence and permanence of heroin addiction.

Concepts of Drug Dependence

In order to treat a problem, there must be some understanding of its underlying nature. This seems self evident and medical technology effectively deals with medical disorders by examining them, literally under the microscope, and coming up with answers which promote understanding of the causes and consequences of disease. This leads logically to a search for an appropriate treatment to effect a cure. Research and experimentation is continually throwing new light on the problems of malignant disease and there will undoubtedly be more medical successes such as those resulting from the use of drugs to treat young people with Hodgkin's disease and the acute childhood leukemias.

This approach is good clean medicine at its best and therefore enjoys support in the form of research cash, political backing and public interest and goodwill. The tangible evidence of effective drugs and healthy patients freed from disease are enough to perpetuate this support system.

The application of science and technology to behavioural problems has met with limited success. Early in this century, the exponents of psychoanalytical theory promised new insights into the working of the human mind and therefore the control or cure of aberrations thereof. To a large extent this has not occurred and although understanding has often replaced fear and mythology, a true perception of why people do what they do remains elusive. In Western countries, the latter half of the twentieth century has been a time of social revolution and provision of opportunities to improve and develop the structure of society, hopefully eliminating for ever such social evils as starvation, hopeless poverty, destitution and homelessness. Although the welfare state has many problems and inequalities, and the delivery of care is inconsistent, much has been achieved.

In recent years a new health initiative has arisen. The new move is based on the assumption that disease may have origins in behaviour which can be avoided. This attractive idea of prevention definitely has appeal and therefore has a large and dedicated following, jogging, eating and thinking their way to longevity. Whether it stands the test of time remains to be seen but it has the added and thoroughly modern attraction of being self determined and free.

Cynics would say that public attitudes are a product of propaganda, or at least of political systems, but nevertheless they are vital in the influence they have over many things, not least disease. The notion that one disease may be a good one and another a bad one seems ridiculous. There are, however, socially acceptable diseases and those which are not referred to in polite society. Those obviously enjoying public sympathy tend to be acute, non-infectious and not causing mental consequences such as confusion or loss of inhibitions. Thus someone with a broken arm or leg, or even a fractured skull, often gets more sympathy than a case of tuberculosis or chronic dementia. This may be a hangover from previous centuries. The idea of mental illness and infectious disease being unclean or visitations from God may be modified in modern society but not totally lost.

Drug dependence has some areas of social acceptability and others of undoubted stigma. To be dependent on cigarettes or alcohol is acceptable, within limits, but dependence on other drugs is not. Even without the associations of crime and corruption, attitudes in many parts of society to a comparatively harmless drug such as cannabis are severe and definite. Illicit drugs as a group, and dependence on them, rate very low in the table of social acceptability. This has its logic when one recognizes the crime and violence associated with the heroin or cocaine trade, but also has its contradictions when the undoubted evils of these people are transferred to the 'street addict'.

The 'soldiers' disease' of the American Civil War, which was a profound addiction to the morphine used at that time for injuries, was as much a 'good disease' as that resulting from the large scale sale of opiate-based proprietary medicines well into this century.

Somehow the tide of public sympathy has been turned against dependence problems and the combined forces of political, public and professional opinion have identified dependence on 'drugs' as not so much a nasty disease as a deadly sin.

All this is an important preamble to discussion about concepts of addiction. Reality may well be a combination of facts and how they are perceived, and in this case the facts are thin on the ground and perception is distorted by a barrage of newspaper headlines, political hyperbole and fear of the unknown.

Alcohol – Addiction or Dependence?

A study of the information available about addiction to any substance inevitably leads to the alcohol story. Probably the first drug to be recognized as causing this type of problem, the idea of alcohol addiction first emerged at the end of the eighteenth century, well before opium was considered in the same light. Since that time it has led the field in Western society and today, in numbers of individuals affected and illness resulting, it is by far the most important drug of abuse. In the 1950s the term addiction came under scrutiny and its limitations were debated. The concept of alcohol addiction as a disease became popular in that decade and it was included in the International Classification of Diseases. At the end of the 1960s the World Health

Organization was again wrestling with the underlying implications of the terms addiction, dependence and disease when applied to a behavioural disorder. The definition which resulted from their deliberations recognized the physical side of the problem but more importantly stressed the psychological nature of the disorder. Most importantly, the definition was inclusive of all drugs and therefore recognized the similarities in behaviour in those abusing a wide variety of substances. The substance itself therefore becomes less important and the behaviour the common theme. The 1969 definition allowed that:

'Drug dependence is a state, psychic and sometimes physical, resulting from the interaction between a living organism and a drug, characterised by behavioural and other responses that always include a compulsion to take the drug on a continuous or periodic basis in order to experience its psychic effects and sometimes to avoid the discomfort of its absence. Tolerance may or may not be present. A person may be dependent on more than one drug.' (WHO, 1969)

This definition included a new term, drug dependence, which for the first time considered features of drugtaking outside the purely physical. The psychological component becomes the main feature and the physical one is not even regarded as always present. Here we must suddenly confront the complexity of the situation, and the idea that regarding drug use as a disease, in the same way as diabetes or coronary heart disease, is inadequate.

Rejection of the Disease Concept of Alcoholism

Following the debate about the nature of alcohol abuse a bit further may be useful in the examination of drugtaking. The use of the term alcohol dependence syndrome in the same way as the WHO definition of drug dependence allows for the physical and psychological components. It does not, however, allow for other factors which many workers consider to be important. Surely social, domestic and environmental factors have some influence on drinking habits and disorders? If they are instrumental in causing alcohol abuse, even in a small way, then the problem may be controlled at least partially by forces outside the individual. In addition, the startlingly obvious observation that many individuals exist in the same environment and with the same pressures without becoming dependent drinkers must be taken into account.

Current Ideas on Alcohol Dependence

These and other debates have given rise to a new pragmatism in the view of alcohol abuse and this in turn has led to some concepts which are designed to be practical rather than clinically precise.

Traditional views of organizations such as Alcoholics Anonymous include the belief that once dependence has been established then absolute abstinence is the only line of management. Increasingly, however, views are being expressed that 'problem drinkers' may return to a normal pattern of drinking and the concept of controlled drinking is one that should be used rather than absolute abstinence. Changing behaviour in order to prevent problem drinking is another area of great current interest and new educational initiatives directed to this end are being pursued with increased confidence. As far as treatment in the traditional sense is concerned, there has been considerable modification in views about how this should be applied to greatest effect. Family therapy and community groups are important innovations and the application of treatment in the home environment, recognizing the importance of this as a causative factor, is a way of providing more effective therapy.

Implications for Therapy

The sometimes tedious and semantic discussions of those interested in alcohol abuse may appear to be irrelevant to the management of those suffering from the disorder. In the same way, the complex and occasionally vituperative debates over definitions and distinctions often seem to cloud the whole issue rather than making it clearer. The passage of time has, however, highlighted the inadequacy of previous concepts and the failure of treatments based on these. Treating alcoholism as a disease has been a manifest failure, as the social, domestic, environmental and other factors are not taken into account. Therapy therefore has moved from the type delivered by a doctor to a patient in a hospital bed to that delivered in the usual environment of the individual by a trained professional. This person may be medically qualified or not, and the therapy may well be unrecognizable as medical treatment; certainly it rarely has much to do with tablets, medicines and the usual idea of cure.

Finally these new approaches have brought with them a move to reduce intervention. This may look like a way out of using resources and time but the concept of 'minimal intervention' currently has many advocates. There is some evidence for the existence of large groups of potential abusers who change their behaviour in a positive direction because of the presence of treatment possibilities, or the smallest amount of intervention such as attendance at one outpatient appointment, and go on to less harmful behaviour. For them, it is more precisely the prospect of treatment that works. Treatment is composed of many facets, not just a face to face encounter between a doctor and a patient. It should be recognized that many factors and many individuals, both professional and non-professional, are involved in altering behaviour.

Heroin Addiction or the Problem Heroin Taker

Can the same evolution be followed for heroin abusers? Certainly progress has been slower and more painful and the disease concept, as applied to heroin users, never managed to convince society that the drug user should be given help in some form or another. This is despite the conclusions of successive British Government Committees which regarded drug use as a medical problem. The US Government reports, specifically the Harrison Act of 1914, however directed that country much more towards the criminal, rather than medical, nature of the phenomenon of opiate abuse.

Perhaps these approaches, in separate ways, have blocked progress in the evolution of a workable concept of dependence as applied to heroin abuse.

Leaving aside legislation and the view of authority on drug abusers, it would be attractive to apply the new directions in alcohol studies to other drugs such as heroin. The substitution of the term problem drugtaker for drug addict is already popular with many of those involved. The use of dependence rather than addiction is also a comparatively new feature which allows us to consider the psychological as well as the physical components of a drug dependence syndrome. The possibility that there may exist a comparable state to controlled drinking in the drug abuser is less popular, but the controlled use of drugs of all sorts undoubtedly exists. Much of the knowledge about what happens to drug users leads to the conclusion that some people become more controlled in their use as time goes on.

The existence of controlled drugtaking is unlikely to be popular with police and political authorities or, for that matter, with the general public, but if it exists then it is futile or even dangerous to ignore it. The general reluctance to accept the patterns of abuse referred to previously are reminiscent of Victorian attitudes to alcoholism and the preference for defining it as a disease. Although attitudes to alcohol have broadened, a narrow line of thinking still persists in other areas of substance abuse.

Drug Dependence Syndrome

The persisting stereotype of the drug 'addict' or 'junkie' in modern times represents perhaps the most determined attempt of society to identify a clear image of heroin takers. The move to the less perjorative term 'dependence' is not so much an attempt to conceal the reality of drug misuse as an attempt to allow a broader understanding of the problem. It helps to separate those heavily and persistently dependent on the drug from those using it intermittently or transitorily. Reluctance to accept this may be a reluctance to admit that heroin use is not associated with intractable dependence or addiction, or a lack of information about the true nature of the dependence process. It may additionally be related to a real and genuine fear that to contemplate heroin use in the absence of 'addiction' is to open the flood gates and experience more widespread use.

Whatever the cause of society's obsession with the term 'addiction', it can be seen that this impedes the ability to cope with the phenomenon in a logical way and may indeed make the situation worse. Drug users themselves are members of society and are therefore subjected to the same information as others. If, then, they believe that addiction is a persisting process then behaviour change is made unnecessarily difficult.

Spontaneous Remission

Longstanding information to counteract the permanence of addiction theory exists in the work of Winick in Seattle and Waldorf in New York. The 'maturing out' hypothesis, which suggests that heroin users stop or modify drug taking behaviour as they grow older, has been supplemented by the information that many do so without any recognized help or treatment. People of any age who have used heroin for a period of time usually attempt, and often succeed in, reducing intake and improving survival chances by modifying damaging behaviour. Bucknall and Robertson in the UK and Zinberg in the US have drawn attention to the large numbers of non-dependent or controlled users who exist in any community and to the suggestion that many more individuals exist for whom heroin use presents no problem which requires specialist help.

Without doing any more research, therefore, we can outline the existing state of affairs amongst heroin users. Most heroin users start taking the drug between 17 and 24 years of age. As an associated feature, but not necessarily because of it, they use other drugs (see Table 1.1).

In the majority of those taking it, heroin use is periodic and decreases as time goes by. Many do not become ill and do not come in contact with the law, the medical profession or the social services. Many use small quantities of heroin and therefore, technically, are not dependent on the drug. Much of the damage arising from heroin use is consequent on its illegal status and the secret and covert nature of its use. Following on from this is the failure of heroin users to understand the dangers or to have access to materials or methods of improving such practices. Without therefore ignoring the dangers and damage caused by heroin, some idea of the variability of problems and the individuality of drug takers can be seen.

Persisting Myths or Illusions

To those engaged in the study of heroin use, the false notion of 'addiction' has long since been discounted. Observations have been made over prolonged periods of individual behaviour which dispel the idea that addiction is

Table 1.1   *Drugs used before and after first heroin use (total number interviewed – 54)*   Source: Bucknall & Robertson, 1986

Drug		Before (%)		After (%)	
Alcohol		51	(94)	53	(98)
Cigarettes		48	(89)	53	(98)
Cannabis		44	(81)	52	(96)
Solvents		21	(39)	23	(43)
Barbiturates		13	(24)	22	(41)
Stimulants:	Amphetamines	12	(22)	41	(76)
	Cocaine	2	(4)	22	(41)
Hallucinogens:	LSD	8	(15)	25	(46)
	Psilocybin	2	(4)	2	(4)
Opiates:	Dihydrocodeine	6	(11)	43	(80)
	Dipipanone	4	(7)	29	(54)
	Morphine	1	(2)	5	(9)
	Buprenorphine	0	(0)	18	(33)
	Dextromoramide	0	(0)	1	(2)
	Methadone	0	(0)	1	(2)
	Opium	0	(0)	1	(2)
Benzodiazepines:	Diazepam	3	(6)	26	(48)
	Nitrazepam	0	(0)	2	(4)
	Triazolam	0	(0)	2	(2)
	Temazepam	0	(0)	1	(2)

a necessary consequence of heroin use. Dependence undoubtedly exists but, as will be seen later, is not always present in heroin users. The permanence of dependence has also been largely disproved and many heroin users abstain on an apparently permanent basis after short or long periods of heroin use. Those who continue may change their type of behaviour, still indulging in drugtaking but in a more controlled and less damaging way both physically and socially. The continuous nature of heroin use is a further area which requires clarification. The contention that heroin users indulge on a continuous basis is questioned by the findings of Robins regarding American military personnel returning from Vietnam. Given the option of abstaining or remaining in Asia, the former state was rapidly attained and subsequently maintained in the majority. At follow-up some years later, a significant percentage, 20%, had used heroin since and 12% were considered to be dependent. In the UK, Bucknall and Robertson have shown that abstinence is a common feature in heroin users, but that even after periods of 12 months the relapse rate is large.

The picture emerging is of a behaviour which is reversible, sometimes permanently, but which is certainly not inevitable or continuous.

The idea that dependent opiate use exists has much support. In a way similar to the ideas now commonplace about alcohol, Zinberg has identified the importance of the drug, the set (that is the individual), the setting and the attitudes and actions of society which influence drugtaking behaviour. He has tried to tease apart these separate factors which go to make up the drug user and to show that all these are required to establish a heroin taker. Close analysis of each component gives an insight into the make-up that initiates and perpetuates this behaviour.

Bucknall and Robertson have attempted to show that heroin use is intermittent and variable in a group of drug users and in each individual case. Over a period of years, most heroin users were found to have periods of re-mission, often prolonged. Only 5% were found to portray the stereotype of a constantly using heroin 'addict', whereas the remainder showed episodes of behaviour change every 5–6 months. Of particular interest and importance was the finding that, as time increases from the onset of use, episodes of abstinence also increase. Large numbers were found to indulge in 'controlled heroin use' and about 5% were 'experimenters', never exhibiting drugtaking behaviour which could be considered to be dependent or extensive.

Zinberg, Bucknall and others conclude from their own researches and from reviewing that of others that not all heroin users become dependent in any physical or psychological way. They also point to the lack of information about this group and how it is likely to be larger than generally identified from studies of groups attending hospital facilities. Many people may pass rapidly in and out of heroin use without detection.

Information Required

Throughout the following chapters it is hoped that the perspectives pre-sented will give rise to questions in the mind of the reader. By pointing out the inadequacy of our current reaction to aspects of the drug problem, it is hoped that the reader will understand why this has been so unsuccessful. An example of this is the failure of treatment for heroin misuse. In the minds of the public is an awareness that some treatment is available and that this may or may not be successful for an individual drug user. Additionally there is an awareness that there is a problem of availability of treatment and that the rich and famous can afford expensive and presumably highly effective therapies, such as acupuncture or neuroelectric therapy, from skilled doctors.

The reality, however, is somewhat different. Treatments proposed and results claimed are enormously confusing. Scientifically, few types of ther-apy have been shown to be highly successful, if the aim is total abstinence. Most claims for substantial 'cures' are based on inadequate data and when scrutinized closely are often misleading and sometimes frankly fraudulent. There is no cure for problems such as drug dependence, any more than there is a single cure for cigarette smoking; some people stop and perhaps more importantly some people reduce their intake to a less damaging level.

For many aspects of the heroin problem we have no answers and, worryingly, professionals and public often behave as if there are enormous amounts of established facts about heroin users and their habits. Despite the widely held view, there is little evidence that all heroin users take increasing amounts of the drug over a period of years or that the majority die quickly of drug related problems. Research into the efficacy of treatment of any sort is conflicting and there is even evidence that some types of treatment may retard a natural recovery process.

The responses by governments and professionals to drug related problems over the last 50 years have tended to be radical and based on an emotional response to a crisis. For this reason sudden changes in attitudes, or the adoption of radical new policies, have obscured the underlying pattern of events and have obstructed the ability to evaluate or assess new policies. The dramatic change from community management of drug problems in the 1960s to specialist units prescribing methadone obscured the underlying behaviour of drug use.

Ten years later the problem had become one of ex-drug users dependent on methadone. The response in the 1980s to a new and larger wave of heroin use throughout the UK was to obtain maximum control by increased criminalization of heroin and heroin use. By a radical change of policy, drug users were pushed from their status as medically dependent to that of criminals, alienated from society. This, remember, happened in the space of a few short years. Appropriate disillusionment with the role of the drug dependency treatment clinics did not give rise to the logical and scientifically based evolution of a new type of management. Instead, society turned its back on a generation of young people and their families, failing to offer even sympathy, far less support. The affluent can at least escape to the Harley Street specialist where sympathy is available, and is perhaps the most effective part of therapy. The not so fortunate are rejected as incurable and often end up in prison.

A failure to respond to the prescriptions of the 1970s has been punished by a backlash of an impatient society.

Prejudice and Fear

Fear of drug users is not a new experience for society but is increasingly apparent, probably because of the increasing numbers of those reported to be taking drugs. Stories of 'crazed dope fiends' were prevalent in the 1960s when all sorts of violent and antisocial acts were attributed to the effects of such mind altering drugs as LSD, cannabis and heroin. Although to a large extent these have been discredited as being inaccurate, fear persists and a genuine belief that loss of inhibitions leads to aggression and violence which are the hallmarks of drug misuse is still commonplace.

Similar problems existed after the use of cannabis (marijuana) became widespread in the 1960s and early 1970s. Such inaccuracies, designed to increase prejudice and fear, were evident in the popular press and the following extract from the Narcotics and Hallucinogens Handbook in 1967 demonstrates this:

> 'Marijuana . . . disrupts and destroys the brain and distorts the mind resulting in crime and degeneracy. It . . . like cocaine is the immediate and direct cause of the crime committed . . . whisky intensifies its violent properties . . .
>
> A person under the influence of marijuana is very dangerous and great caution must be used in effecting his arrest.
>
> The great danger of this drug is the general release of inhibitions accompanied by a diminution or loss of moral sense. The user is very often dangerous to handle or control, has no fear, feels no pain, and many commit crimes of violence.' (J. B. Williams (Ed.))

Despite the subsequent reports in the US of the National Commission on Marijuana and Drug Abuse (1971) and in the UK of the Advisory Council on the Misuse of Drugs (1969), which both concluded that there was no evidence to substantiate any of these claims, the web of anxiety is difficult to unravel even years after the scientific realities emerged. This sort of information, therefore, is not based so much on facts as on a situation distorted by prejudice and fear. Such an account has the double effect of reinforcing the anxieties which society properly has about drug taking and further alienating those taking the drug.

Prejudice based on fear is in turn based on inaccurate or insufficient knowledge. Individuals who have experienced drugs are unlikely to admit this to others even though their experience may not be comparable with that of the common beliefs.

A situation has arisen now that is self-perpetuating. Because of our prejudice against drug users and our fear of drugs, we are unable to see the true reality of the situation. Instead of adolescents with problems, we see demons and criminals. Those who have a controlled or non-problematic pattern of drug use remain undetected and the stereotype occupies the attention of the public and the limelight in the media. Our failure to see beyond the web of anxieties obscures our vision of the problem and does an injustice to those involved. Not only that, it prevents any progression to more appropriate means of control and treatment.

The failure of medicine and society to be consistent and rational has allowed a situation in which there is much uncertainty about the real truths and facts. Drugtakers and society are no longer clear about the dangers and risks of drug taking and as a state of confusion and anxiety increases, the very real dangers are overlooked or ignored.

Society's Need for a Cure

Perhaps one of the reasons why society regards heroin use as intractable is the failure to find a cure that can be applied in a uniform and effective way. The phenomenon of heroin use undoubtedly presents enormous problems for all of us in economic, medical and social contexts. The acceptance that opiate use is variable, sometimes transitory and usually changing, often for the better, with time, takes away the need to search for a cure. There can be no single or simple cure for a complex of social, personal, domestic and environmental problems.

As we will examine later, the concept of cure may be behind much of the confusion. Drug use is, most of the time, not an all-or-nothing phenomenon but a situation of enormously variable severity. It varies in individuals over a period of time and there are enormous differences in types and consequences of drug use between different individuals.

Faced with a media report, therefore, of the 'drug addiction' of a personality or pop star, conclusions should not be drawn without further information. The individual, the type of drug or drugs used, the length of time the drugtaking has gone on, the personal situation and problems associated with the drug taken are all pieces of information which should be acquired before the true problem can be assessed. In the perspective of his or her social situation and various pressures existing in their lives, a different reality may emerge which has little to do with drugs. Faced with the same individual and the revelation that he or she is an adolescent or is undecided about his or her future or even that, through poor advice, is bankrupt, the cry would not be for a cure but for support, advice and a chance to re-evaluate themselves.

Society feels it needs, deserves and therefore demands a cure or a solution to the perceived problem. Perhaps that perception is creating the problem or at least adding to it.

Recovery or Cure

Against the background of confusion, most of all about the nature of drug dependence, there is a further illusion. This is that there is such a thing as a cure for all dependent people. Despite the increasing awareness of drug use as a behavioural phenomenon rather than a disease, the idea that treatment is available and effective persists. This is of course a false idea and, as will be examined more closely in a later chapter, treatment should properly be directed at predisposing factors related to drugtaking, if these exist, and the damaging consequences of the habit. The best treatment is prevention of drugtaking.

The notion of cure or even therapy in a condition characterized by its variability is inappropriate, as is that of recovery. When has recovery been achieved? In the case of a broken leg, is it when the patient leaves hospital with a plaster of Paris, or is it when the leg is functioning normally again? If a residual limp is present is recovery complete, partial or adequate? The recovering drugtaker in a similar way may exhibit partial, incomplete or temporary recovery. He may indeed continue to use drugs on a rare occasion in a manner causing no apparent damage to himself or others. His recovery may or may not be adequate in this case. Society must consider these questions.

As in the recovery from alcoholism, a decision has to be made as to what situation one will accept. Complete, absolute and permanent abstention from the drug is the ideal, but does one drink imply that all is lost or one shot of heroin a wasted attempt at therapy? Clearly if some improvement is visible or damage averted, then something has been achieved.

If the 'recovered' drug user has the occasional lapse into heroin use but meanwhile maintains his occupational, social and domestic responsibilities, then recovery must be at least as impressive as the limping individual who had a broken leg. Recovery as a concept must be qualified and claims for treatment must be related to their ability to effect long term change.

This leads to difficulties in assessing treatment and agencies providing assistance. If, as suspected, changes occur over a period of time, regardless of experience with treatment, then how can the value of treatment be assessed? If therapy in, for example, a residential establishment takes two years, or a drug user is in goal for a similar period, is it the passage of time or the experience of treatment or incarceration which accounts for any change observed later?

Attitudes of Society

The development of complex social mechanisms for the use of those drugs which are legal, such as alcohol, cigarettes and prescribed drugs, is in contrast with those that have been regarded as unacceptable and therefore made illegal, such as cannabis, cocaine and heroin. The fact that these legal drugs would be unlikely to pass the test of acceptability if newly available today is not meant to imply that legalization of heroin would solve any problems; it would not. It indicates however that there is a certain inconsistency, not to say hypocrisy, in our attitudes to different drugs.

Opiate users therefore have traditionally been regarded as socially outcast and dealt with by criminal and legal means rather than medical or social constraints. The alcohol abuser, however, is comparatively acceptable even though the cost to society in terms of health and damage to innocent people is much greater. Moreover, in the UK the view that drug use is a criminal activity is increasing and almost 5,000 individuals received custodial sentences for drug offences in 1984 (21% more than in 1983). The proportional use of custody for unlawful possession of cannabis was 13% even though this drug has never been shown to have the serious health consequences of cigarettes, alcohol and some prescribed drugs.

Clearly there is a problem here not related to medicine but to social control and public acceptability. Such policies are undoubtedly popular as evidenced by the support given to them by the voter at election time. This is understandable, we are all interested in the future of society and recognize that if it is to run well and to the advantage of the majority, then there must be constraints on some members. The time has come however to look carefully at drugs and drugtakers and consider whether or not we can afford to continue with our present views and attitudes.

Good Drugs and Bad Drugs

Largely for reasons of control and prevention of use, drugs are seen by society as those which are legal and available and therefore 'good', and those which are illegal and not widely available and therefore 'bad'. In the context of law and order and the maintenance of social control, this is straightforward and acceptable. However it takes no account of the paradox which exists when one considers the damage done by drugs in these different categories. The destructive effect on health and social damage stems largely from the use of 'good' drugs. The expense incurred by the use of 'bad' drugs stems largely from the cost of implementing control and constraint over those involved. Cigarettes accounted for an estimated 100,000 premature deaths in the UK in 1986 and there were 18,000 hospital admissions for alcohol related disorders. In addition there were 226,000 convictions for drunkenness offences. Research has demonstrated that 96% of the population use alcohol.

In a recent study at Oxford University in a population aged 18–20 years, more than 10% of a group of 178 students were found to have used benzodiazepine drugs, that is prescribed tranquillizing drugs like Valium, Librium or Ativan. National figures show an annual provision of 13 million prescriptions for drugs in this category. Increasingly there is an awareness of the dangers and side effects of these drugs and Ashton has suggested that they may cause dependence and possibly lasting damage to brain tissue when used over long periods of time. The effects of withdrawal are often confused with the original anxiety which initiated treatment and continued and increasing use results.

The paradox is that 'bad' drugs such as heroin, cocaine and cannabis produce no such tissue damage, and problems arising from their use stem mainly from their illegal status and subsequent impurity, contamination and septic use.

Requirements for Information

Although much is understood about drug misuse and those taking drugs, for many reasons various myths and misconceptions are perpetuated. Many of the possible causes and associations with use are politically sensitive and connections with poor housing, poverty, unemployment and disillusionment are unlikely to be popular messages for any government. It is much easier to see it in black and white, namely, drug users are criminals and non drug users are not, rather than to address the complex underlying issues.

Politicians will look for a policy to pursue with drug users, police will look for convictions of those involved and doctors will look for a cure for the disease and all will continue to be disappointed until the underlying problems are considered and the preconceived ideas are dispelled. To this end much information is required and to a certain extent social change is mandatory.

Little is understood about the day to day activities of drug users in terms of quantities of drug taken. Nothing substantial is recorded about those who use the drug intermittently. Many have taken heroin, even intravenously, once or twice and then never again. Large numbers of drugtakers stop using heroin with no treatment and remain abstinent. Even longstanding abusers go through phases of heavy use and prolonged phases of light or 'non-dependent' use. Lastly, many illegal heroin users continue over a period of decades and remain fit. Good examples of the non-damaging effects of opiates are the longstanding attenders of maintenance clinics where, over many years, they have taken much larger quantities of drugs than their contemporaries who rely on the illegal sources, the drug in this case usually being methadone.

Conventional wisdom maintains that heroin users are responsible for much crime in Western society. Does this mean that all heroin users indulge in criminal behaviour? Some problem drinkers do, but not all. Some cigarette smokers are criminals but not all. Certainly the illegal status of heroin makes a user by definition a criminal, but is enough known about the behaviour of heroin users and the illegal market to assume that each individual is inflicting more damage on society than a drunken driver or even a sober driver exceeding the speed limit?

Finally, the social position of the heroin user makes it difficult to form a clear picture of what happens. If he or she dies, then this fact appears as a statistic in the appropriate column and even then there is a bias. The knowledge of heroin use in an individual dying of other causes may influence these statistical records in a way that legal drug use such as alcohol or cigarettes might not. For example death from pneumonia in a drug user may be attributed to opiate abuse, where it might not paradoxically be attributed to chronic cigarette consumption.

The drug user remaining fit and active is likely to be able to conceal his illegal activity. Furthermore those experiencing long term abstinence and more conventional social activity are unlikely to draw attention to previous behaviour. Information therefore is sparse concerning the longevity and social activity of the growing numbers of individuals in contemporary society who have used heroin in the past. The acquisition of this information is important not only to the understanding of the nature of the problem but to its treatment.

Society Reinforces Addiction

Classical psychological theory gives us the concept of operant conditioning which describes how behaviour is modified in either a positive or negative way by rewards or punishments. Thus behaviour which results in a reward is more likely to be repeated and that which results in a negative experience is less likely to be repeated.

Used as a theory for behavioural disorders this has some application in day to day management of such disorders as anxiety and phobias. For the drug user however, alienated from society, rejected by family and punished at every opportunity in his or her contact with agencies such as those enforcing the law, it would seem that powerful conditions exist to discourage antisocial behaviour. There must therefore be factors to counteract this force. Punishment and coercion have never appeared to work well in the control of drug dependence and there are many examples of prohibition tending to encourage use rather than eliminate it. The factors encouraging use and availability must clearly be more powerful than those against. Many economic and commercial forces operate in this field and where there is a market for a substance, be it a drug or a washing powder, a mechanism will exist to supply that commodity. If, however, there are such powerful forces operating to discourage drugtaking then one might expect its use to diminish. The factors promoting its use must be carefully considered as these must be equally motivating if they are to counterbalance the social disapproval, the legal constraints, the possibility of penal detention and the dangers of physical injury or harm. Having failed to control or eradicate the two ends of the drug use problem, availability and demand, by conventional means such as legal control and social disapproval, the understanding of the conditions which encourage continued use and which stimulate the desire to try a new experience with psychoactive substances becomes crucially important. If the present trend of increasing numbers of young people using drugs is to be reversed, then a knowledge of the factors that encourage it is a good starting point.

Why Do People Take That First Shot?

Self reported answers to this question from many groups of drug users fail to identify any one single motivating factor which causes the initiation into drug use of any sort. Most individuals will say that they were interested to try a new experience, they were bored at the time and wanted some excitement, companions were doing it or they did it without thinking very much about it, because it was there. It does seem, however, that availability, curiosity, peer group pressure, boredom and the awareness of social disapproval or physical danger are all factors which cause an individual to try a drug. Thus at this stage there is not usually a positive effort to identify a place where the drug can be found and a time which might be suitable, but rather a combination of coincidences which lead to a situation in which, for all these reasons, it is difficult to refuse the offer. Many say that they lacked the information at the time to resist these pressures. Often they did not know what type of drug they were taking and only later realized that it was heroin or cocaine.

Having used a drug once does not mean that the dependence is established. This is true of heroin as it is of any substance and the majority of those who experiment with alcohol or even cigarettes do not become dependent in any sense after their first or even many experiences. However, continued use depends very much on that first experience or on the early pattern of use. If this is pleasurable then it is more likely to be repeated and if repeated exposure is again rewarded by positive feelings and associations then further use will follow. One thing known about opiates is that they induce a sense of wellbeing, a sort of detached contentment and a release from the cares and worries of the present. This may be especially useful in the presence of pain but in the presence of mental anguish it is likely to be equally effective. The contented, fit, healthy adolescent with prospects of employment and the stimulus of a prosperous and fulfilling future is therefore unlikely to be in need of such a release. The unemployed socially deprived youngster with a poor educational record and limited prospects, however, might find a stimulating alternative in heroin use as a release from perpetual social pressures and unfulfillable temptations. The further into the social trap one sinks, the more attractive is the admittedly short term solution of heroin.

The use of a drug as an escape from reality need not necessarily apply only to the socially disadvantaged, and heroin use is not confined to one single group. It is not difficult to imagine a situation in other sectors of society in which such pressures exist, leading to the requirement for a means to break out or establish an alternative lifestyle.

To understand the initial attraction to heroin use should not therefore be impossible, and the way in which society can precipitate such a situation in a young person is something which must be grasped. If a pattern has been established in the life of an individual which has precipitated heroin use then it is something which requires more than casual recognition. Something or a number of things have led to this and although it is agreed below that these may be quite benign and the situation may reverse spontaneously or with minimal intervention, in other cases the die may already be cast. In many cases the use of drugs appears inevitable and the attraction to illegal activities or entertainments is evident from an early age. Thus an individual from a broken home with experience of parental addiction or instability and with a fragmented educational background might be at greater risk than an individual with a more stable childhood.

Heroin, or other drugtaking, may be motivated by many factors. It has many ingredients to satisfy the urgent requirements of adolescence or early adult life. It encompasses excitement, fear, risk, intense emotional experience and close group identification. It represents for many an escape from problems or a reality which seems dull or uninteresting.

Conclusion

There are many unanswered questions about heroin use in the 1980s. The received wisdom of the black and white nature of drugs and the existence of good and bad drugs must now be considered scientifically unacceptable. The heroin user should no longer be regarded as a member of a deviant subgroup as this obscures the reality of many otherwise normal individuals becoming involved with the drug.

Possibly most important, the illusion that heroin use is an irreversible addiction has to be reconsidered. The belief that this is the case makes it more difficult for society to understand the obvious contradictions in this view. Furthermore, the belief is also prevalent amongst those taking heroin, thus obstructing progress to the drug free state. Abstinent heroin users will often state that the turning point only came when they realized that they could stop if they wanted to. False beliefs therefore perpetuate dependence.

The all or nothing view of drug abuse held by society and at times by drugtakers maintains that continued use of heroin or relapse into heroin use represents failure. Progression to a more controlled or less damaging type of drug use is something that is often only apparent to families of drug users or those living close to them. Professionals maintain the all or nothing view and often for this reason fail to observe improvement in behaviour or to encourage gradual change in this direction.

The obsession with total abstinence obscures the possibility that improvement can occur in other ways. Improvement does occur over time and with increased knowledge and information. To allow this improvement should be our major purpose as professionals and as a society.

2 Heroin – The Hard Drug

The position occupied popularly by heroin as the 'hardest drug', and the perception of it as the source of many of the social evils in modern society, depend on many things not necessarily related to its effect on the human body or its properties as a drug of dependence. In common with other social evils there are many facets to heroin use. Many of the problems associated with use of heroin are related to its illegality rather than its toxicity, and its position as a socially unacceptable drug has an important influence on the real and apparent dangers.

History

Opium, the parent compound, is the dried juice from unripe seed capsules of the opium poppy (*Papaver somniferum*), which is indigenous in Asia Minor, but is now widely cultivated. The alkaloids of opium include morphine and codeine and 18 others. Heroin or diamorphine is derived from morphine and is prepared by an acetylation process. This was first done in 1874, and diamorphine was introduced as a remedy for coughs and paradoxically as a treatment for morphine addiction.

Morphine, derived from opium, was well known in ancient times and was used as far back as 4000 BC for its psychological effects as well as a powerful pain relieving compound. In Greek and Roman civilizations it was used as a sleeping draught and this use persisted in Europe into the early part of the twentieth century. Arab physicians in ancient times were well versed in the use of opium and introduced the drug to the Orient, where it was largely used for treating dysentery.

In the sixteenth century, Paracelsus (1493–1541), the Swiss physician, gave the name Laudanum (from the Latin *laudare* – to praise) to preparations of opium, and about 1680 Thomas Sydenham introduced it to Britain. In the East, British and French colonization created problems when in 1840 the Chinese Emperor, Tao Kaung, tried to impose restrictions on opium smoking, which by then had increased to enormous proportions. The subsequent Opium Wars (1839–1842 and 1856), in which the British were victorious, saw the increase in opium trade between India and China, greatly increasing the size of the problem. At the end of the first Opium War, the Treaty of Nanking agreed that the British took possession of Hong Kong and were allowed unlimited importation of opium to China. At that time official recognition of this trade as an important source of revenue was undoubtedly the reason for official approval which continued well into the present century.

Societies for social reform and recognition of the problems caused by these policies encountered an uphill struggle for many decades. In a similar pattern today, but without the sanction of governments, the economy of the drug trade is the single most important factor in its continued strength. When profits are so large, business will continue and the windfall nature of the income at every level ensures a continuing number of willing suppliers. The underlying stimulus to the trade is therefore greed and power, a similar situation today in the West to that 100 years ago in the East.

In 1803, a German pharmacist called Serturner isolated the alkaloid which he called Morphia (after Morpheus the Greek god of dreams). Heroin was first produced in the United Kingdom in 1893, almost 100 years after morphine was derived as the major active ingredient of opium. Its value over morphine as a pain killing drug is still the subject of debate, but its conversion to morphine in the bloodstream means that, at least if taken by the oral or inhalation routes, the effects are very similar. If injected, however, the quantity of heroin reaching the brain is increased and the effect is more profound. The greater ability of heroin to penetrate the brain is established as the main reason for its increased activity as a pain killer or psychoactive agent. Its administration by injection therefore makes it a particularly powerful agent.

Recent historical events, giving rise to the present international drugs trade, have reflected a different pattern in different Western European and North American countries. State control over prescribing and legislation on medical use of various drugs gave rise to a different manifestation of the problem in separate countries. Over the last decade, however, these differences are disappearing and a similar pattern is developing in many countries. This has come about perhaps as the illegal trade becomes more sophisticated and modern technology allows easier and less controlled travel. Variations in legal controls have tended to disappear and the 'British system' of provision of heroin to those addicted has given way to a pattern more in common with the United States. This change may have been as a result of changing patterns of heroin use, but whatever the cause it is unlikely that such a system could have resisted the influx of large quantities of high purity heroin from the Middle East in the late 1970s and early 1980s. The prospect of treating the large number of heroin users now reported from most centres in the UK by this type of provision is less than realistic. Moreover, the concept of treatment by substitution therapy may, for many reasons explained later, be more likely to create long term problems than effect cure in the short term.

In many countries the drug problem therefore follows a similar pattern. As far as heroin is concerned the preference for intravenous use gives rise to the most dramatic and damaging manifestations of drug misuse and perhaps the most important long term consequences, namely the spread of bloodborne virus infections such as AIDS and hepatitis.

United States of America

The invention of the hypodermic syringe in 1853, shortly before the American Civil War (1861–1865), led to enormous use of morphine for battle injuries. So much so that morphine dependence became so common as to be called the 'soldier's disease'. Subsequent rapid growth of the population of the United States, and comparatively poor provision of medical services, led to an enormous use of patent medicines, many containing opiates. By the latter half of the nineteenth century, an estimated 4% of the population were regular users and 0.25% were thought to be opiate dependent. In the 1890s, with the situation aggravated by the introduction of heroin as a therapy, the seriousness of the situation was becoming apparent. A tax on opium was introduced in 1890, followed by total prohibition in 1909.

The Harrison Act (or Narcotic Act) of 1914 was the first major piece of legislation and established the trend which has continued in America to the present day. The use of drugs covered by the Act was permitted for medical purposes, but the treatment of opiate dependence was not regarded as a legitimate medical use. Many physicians were prosecuted and imprisoned for prescribing in this way. The large numbers of opiate users, at that time estimated to be between 200,000 and one million, suddenly became dependent on the illegal market to obtain supplies of opiates.

Heroin or diacetylmorphine (known in Britain as diamorphine) became the main drug of use and its production, importation and use was banned completely in 1925. The Narcotics Control Act of 1956 further increased the criminalization of diacetylmorphine and there was established a severe mandatory sentencing policy for those convicted of its possession or use. Minimum sentences of two years for first offence, five years for second and ten years for third were established. Sale of the substance to a minor was punished by life imprisonment or death.

Despite these increasingly punitive measures, the numbers of drug users continued to increase over the next few decades.

In 1968, the control centre was changed from the Bureau of Internal Revenue to the Bureau of Narcotics and Dangerous Drugs of the Department of Justice. The policy however of regarding non-medical use of drugs, including heroin, other opiates, cocaine, cannabis and psychedelics, as criminal behaviour continued.

Throughout the twentieth century the numbers of people using heroin has increased. Roughly 0.1% of the entire population were estimated to be habitual users of heroin in the late 1960s.

The introduction of large scale methadone treatment programmes was the next major step in the attempt to control use or provide therapy. Methadone is a synthetic opiate with properties differing from heroin or morphine which make it a useful alternative. Later on, the effectiveness of this treatment in the 1970s and 1980s will be examined.

United Kingdom

As in America, the widespread use and availability of opiate-containing remedies led to substantial dependence problems by the end of the nineteenth century. The Dangerous Drugs Act of 1920 imposed control over importation and restriction of use of opium products. However, there was little control over medical use of opiates and this was further approved by the Rolleston Committee in 1926, when they reviewed the 1920 Act. The contrast between the medicalization of dependence in the UK and the criminalization of opiate use in the USA was a major feature of this legislation.

Only in 1954 did the Home Office begin to regard and record heroin use as a separate category from other illicit drug use and then there were only 57 individuals known to be dependent on opiates. At that time they were largely 'therapeutic addicts' (dependent by virtue of receiving opiates for legitimate pain relief), and some medical and professional workers with access to pharmaceutical supplies. Illegal sources were almost unknown.

By 1960, there were 94 known heroin users and 175 by 1962. In 1964, there were still only 342. In the mid 1960s, the numbers began to increase fairly rapidly and a new body (the Brain Committee) convened twice, in 1961 and 1965, to review the Dangerous Drugs Act. The conclusion of the first committee was a complacent assumption that problems of heroin use were small and therefore the system was adequate. The conclusion of the 1965 report was that a few physicians were responsible for massive inappropriate prescribing, and led to restriction of prescribing to registered medical practitioners at special centres, and that dependent persons be notified on a central register held at the Home Office. The Misuse of Drugs Act (1971) made more general provision for control and prosecution of drug offenders and also established the Advisory Council on the Misuse of Drugs, which was set the task of keeping under review the misuse of drugs in the UK and advising ministers on measures to deal with problems.

In 1968 centres throughout the UK were designated as drug dependence clinics. Successes, measured by improved behaviour and abstinence, were notable in both Britain and the USA with initial populations treated with methadone as a substitute for heroin. This led to the further enthusiastic supply of funds to develop, especially in the USA, places for all those using heroin. As time went by such enthusiasm was replaced by a more critical evaluation of success and latterly disillusionment, especially in the UK, on the part of both medical supervisors and patients. In Britain, after ten years of clinic availability, the system has finally been swept from its unsteady foundations by the rapid increase of those using heroin in the early 1980s.

Pharmacology

Analgesics, or pain killers, are subdivided into various groups of which the opiates, or narcotic analgesics, are those with morphine-like effects. These are widely and successfully used in the management of severe and intractable pain. The presence of a feeling of wellbeing and euphoria with relief of tension is a major advantage in treating those dying of a painful condition, or suffering unbearable pain. Opiates are all central nervous system depressants. They suppress the cough reflex, interfere with respiration, stimulate the vomiting reflex and increase smooth muscle tone and this gives rise to some unwanted side-effects even in therapeutic doses. These side-effects, however, can be utilized for cough, diarrhoea or acute pain.

Many factors can modify the response of the body to narcotic analgesics and there are many situations in which it is dangerous to use such a drug; the elderly or the young, those with impaired liver capability lacking the normal ability to metabolize the drug, and those with compromised respiratory function are all more susceptible to side-effects. Those patients with head injury or unconsciousness due to ingestion of other drugs may be in danger from the effects of narcotic drugs. The central nervous system depressant effect of a narcotic combined with alcohol, sedatives, hypnotics, tranquillizers, antihistamines or anaesthetic agents may cause serious respiratory depression leading to death from asphyxia.

Opioids, Pain Killers and Related Drugs

The confusing area of terminology relating to this group of drugs arises from the ever increasing numbers of similar chemicals now identified. Terms such as narcotic, opiate, morphine-like drugs and others are often used interchangeably and new drugs with different properties are often referred to as if they had the same effects on the body. The discovery of natural substances existing in the normal body tissues which have opiate properties has aroused much interest but the three groups, *enkephalins*, *endorphins* and *dynorphins* have actions and properties which are far from clear.

The division of the opiates into three categories has some advantages in understanding how they are related. First, drugs with primarily morphine-like effects, opium, heroin and morphine itself; second, those like naloxone

(Narcan) with directly antagonistic effects; and third, those like nalorphine, pentazocine (Fortral) and buprenorphine (Temgesic), which have both types of action.

Heroin

Heroin is two to three times as potent as morphine on a weight to weight basis, and it is commonly thought to produce a greater degree of analgesia with fewer adverse effects. There is, however, little convincing evidence that this is so and this is reflected in the variation in its availability for medical use throughout the world. Heroin is rapidly changed in the body to monoacetyl-morphine and morphine. Its rapid onset of action is attributed to the fat solubility of heroin and monoacetyl-morphine, which allows rapid passage across the so-called blood-brain barrier into the brain tissue where it has its central pain killing activity as well as mood altering effects.

Morphine

This is the main active ingredient of opium and as such is one of the oldest drugs known to humanity. It remains the most commonly legally used narcotic and is the standard drug against which all other analgesics are compared.

Pethidine

This drug is a synthetic pain killer which has many of the actions of morphine although it is not chemically related. It is less likely to cause some of the minor side-effects such as constipation, cough suppression or pupil constriction but, in equivalent doses, has the same analgesic, euphoric, emetic and respiratory depressant activity.

Methadone

Methadone is another synthetic opiate, developed during World War II in Germany and originally called Adolphine after Adolf Hitler. It has similarities to heroin or morphine in terms of its strength of analgesic properties, but it is more effective than these orally and it has a longer duration of action. Methadone is usually effective for 8–12 hours and remains in measurable amounts for much longer. It is an effective cough suppressant and is used for relief of pain in malignant disease.

Its comparatively slow onset of effectiveness when taken by mouth and its relatively slow development of tolerance are major advantages in its use as a treatment for narcotic dependence. The longer action allows for considerably improved control of lifestyle when used under supervision by the heroin

Fig. 2.1 *Relative intensities and time courses of withdrawal reactions after maximum tolerance has been established to each drug*

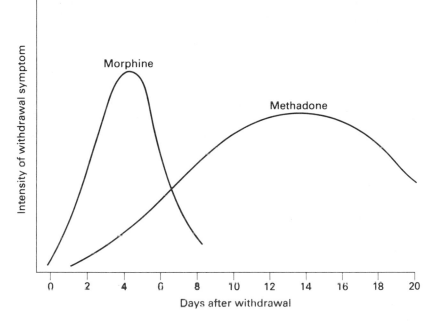

user. The same advantages, however, give rise to problems at a later stage when progression to a drug free state is considered necessary. As can be seen from the graph above, a protracted disappearance from the bloodstream occurs with methadone. This long tail-off in pharmacological activity compares with the rapid disappearance of morphine from the body and may give rise to prolonged symptoms during withdrawal of the drug.

Table 2.1 shows the strength of methadone in comparison with other opiates.

Table 2.1

1 mg methadone equivalent to:	3 mg morphine sulphate
	1 mg heroin
	30 mg codeine
	20 mg pethidine

Codeine and Dihydrocodeine

Both these narcotics have significant effects as analgesics and some effects as cough and respiratory depressants. Their action depends very much on dose and their side-effects are said to be less than the more powerful narcotics. As drugs of abuse, their main dangers lie in their ability to combine with other drugs taken to produce dangerous respiratory depression.

Dextropropoxyphene

Used in combination with paracetamol or asprin or on its own, this drug is marketed under several different names (Doloxene, Darvon, Dolene, Distalgesic, Coproxamol). It is mentioned here because of its opiate-like effects and its toxicity. Comparatively small numbers of tablets can cause respiratory depression and death and in association with other opiates, alcohol, sedatives and paracetamol, toxicity and death are increased.

Partly because of this danger when taken in combination and partly because of its availability and incorrectly assumed safety, this drug accounts for a significant percentage of overdose deaths, accidental or intentional.

Psychopharmacology

Confusion and prejudice dominate all aspects of the understanding of the actions of psychoactive drugs in our society. There are emotions and fears connected with reports of the effects of amphetamines, cannabis, barbiturates, heroin, cocaine and alcohol. 'Miracle' tranquillizers have given way to profound anxiety about the dangers of addiction to or dependence on Ativan, Valium and Librium. The belief that medically prescribed drugs are safe and illicit drugs are dangerous is giving way to general appreciations of the risks and hazards of all psychoactive substances. An inevitable consequence of this is a careful examination of the wisdom of the pharmaceutical industry and the medical profession, as well as close scrutiny of our own personal requirements for treatment based on drugs.

More than 20 years after the explosion in availability of pharmaceutically prepared substances, and after many years of awareness of solvent, LSD, barbiturate and opiate abuse, it is difficult to assess the risks or benefits of such preparations. The ability of such drugs and compounds to alter mood or behaviour remains an elusive quality which has benefits and dangers.

Addiction

The current technical definitions of heroin dependence emphasize the presence of a physical and a psychological component. These two components, along with an understanding of tolerance (a response in the body in recognition of the substance, reducing its action), form the basis of our everyday understanding of drug related problems. The image of clearly defined conditions with measurable levels of severity does not, however, represent the truth. The difficulties in categorizing drug problems and problem drug users has caused a shift away from the term 'addiction' to the wider concepts of dependence. This allows for drug use not connected with obvious physical consequences and includes those opiate, alcohol or substance misusers who are clearly not physically dependent but in a different way experience adverse consequences related to their drug use.

The World Health Organization's Expert Committee on Dependence Producing Drugs has categorized such substances into those producing physical dependence and those producing only psychological dependence. Alcohol and opiates are in both categories, whereas amphetamines, cocaine, cannabis and hallucinogens are said to produce only psychological dependence. Increasingly, however, the emerging information indicates that these effects are not substance specific and that apparent physical effects are present in a wide range of substances from cigarettes to tranquillizers and cocaine.

Work in England (Ashton 1984) has identified a legion of physical effects associated with benzodiazepines, a group of drugs previously thought to have few physical dependence problems. Similarly, many of the physical effects attributed to narcotic withdrawal may be exaggerated by folklore, prejudice and manipulation or connected with consecutive use of excessive quantities of other drugs such as alcohol, tobacco or tranquillizers.

This shift of attention from a specific drug or constellation of symptoms is useful for many reasons. Firstly it draws attention to the individual rather than the drug. Secondly it allows consideration of more than just the withdrawal phase and commits those involved to the longer term nature of the problem. Finally it emphasizes the variability of the effects of drug dependence and the similarities in consequences of different kinds of drugs.

The public and professional understanding of the variability of drug dependence, and the fact that it may be applied to many legal as well as illegal drugs, causes further blurring of the edges of such terms and definitions. The more recent term of 'problem drug use' allows for drug use to exist without the implication of socially or medically damaging consequences. At the same time it suggests that, under certain conditions, almost any substance can become a problem in one way or another. The limitation in this term, however, is defining when use becomes a problem. The user may not perceive it as such and it may only be family, friends or professionals who would consider it to be 'a problem'.

The application of the term addict to an individual, or addiction to the use of a drug, is further confused when the people involved have different ideas of what is meant by that term. Sectors of society have widely differing beliefs about the safety and dangers of drugs and what may be acceptable behaviour to one may be regarded as harmful behaviour by another. This applies to legal as well as illegal drugs. Further, one sector of society may consider another to have a profound need for treatment for this behaviour, even though those taking the drug do not. This is often the situation with heroin use. It is increasingly being used by young people in a way that does not immediately cause problems of a medical or psychiatric nature. Those indulging in its use therefore do not consider it to be a problem and an abstract term like 'addiction' is of little relevance to them. Why, therefore, should they listen to those sectors of society who would change this behaviour without replacing it with any other pleasurable pastime? Pressure to change will be resisted if the motives are suspected and currently the confrontations between heroin user and non-user are increasingly bitter.

Tolerance

In the World Health Organization definition of drug dependence, it is stated that 'tolerance may or may not be present'. It is generally a feature of continued use of opiates that decreased intensity and shortened duration of the analgesic, sedative and euphoric effects develop quickly with repeated dosage.

In medical conditions, 5–10 mg of heroin is usually enough to produce the desired pain killing effect, and the associated relaxation and release from anxiety is usually an additional beneficial feature. In those requiring repeated administration of the drug for ongoing painful conditions the required dose may rapidly rise, 30–40 mg several times a day being easily tolerated and the upper limit being undetermined.

In the use of illegal heroin, amounts used and tolerated by the body are enormously variable and depend much on the regularity with which it is used, the purity of the supply available and the money available to the user to purchase such drugs.

Purities vary from country to country and from city to city, but street level heroin in New York appears to be 5–10% pure, whereas that in British centres is often between 20% and 40% pure.

Franken and Stanwell reported in *The Lancet* in 1961 that they prescribed 1,800 mg of heroin for an individual, per day, in order to 'treat' his heroin dependence problem. Initial experience in the drug dependence clinics were of enormous tolerance developing where supplies were readily available. Gossop (1982) describes a known heroin user taking 1,000 mg of heroin and 600 mg of cocaine during a four hour period under supervision at a clinic.

For the tolerant user, therefore, there is no known upper limit to the amount of drug which can be taken without causing death.

In the non-tolerant user, however, the picture may be quite different. For the individual with no previous experience of heroin taking, those who have been off the drug for long enough for the body to return to the non-tolerant state, and for those taking illicit heroin of an unknown purity, dangers exist with even small doses. A new user may require 5–10 mg and the average daily dose of others may be 80–100 mg. Intakes vary enormously, even in the same person, and during a period of years an individual heroin user may vary from 40–50 mg twice a week to 400 mg per day or more.

Experience in clinics prescribing methadone on a maintenance basis to drug users has shown that tolerance develops to some effects but is incomplete. Thus in addition to constipation, insomnia and decreased sexual function occur in 10–20% of patients and 50% complain of excessive sweating. Maintained on more than 100 mg per day for more than eight weeks, sedation and apathy persist with constricted pupils and decreased respiratory rates (Martin *et al.* 1973). This however can be managed by reduced dosage.

Adulterants in Street Heroin

As will be noted in subsequent chapters on medical problems arising out of illegal heroin use, much of the trouble is caused by contamination of needles and syringes. The material injected is itself far from pure and, unlike a pharmaceutically prepared drug, has no fixed quantity or quality. As the progression from large scale supplier to local user continues, increasing amounts of substances and chemicals are added in order to make what is available go further. Police believe they have found the important suppliers in the distribution hierarchy when quantities seized are large, and when purities are above 50%.

If anything between 50% and 95% of the powder to be injected is not heroin, then its constituents are enormously variable. They often reflect local availability, although some other active ingredients are often present. Quinine is a drug often found in New York heroin, and may be responsible for some side-effects. Cocaine is used in combination with heroin in that city, although to a lesser extent in Europe. Barbiturates, amphetamines, methaqualone (Mandrax), benzodiazepines (Ativan, Valium, Librium) and phenolphthalein are all drugs with an active effect when injected. Phenolphthalein has a laxative effect and may prevent chronic constipation. The effects of the other drugs may account for increased sedation, sudden overdose deaths or other subjective feelings experienced by the user.

The upper limits of tolerance and therefore use have never been established but in controlled clinic situations, individuals have often been known to regularly use the methadone equivalent of 1000–2000 mg daily. The average consumption is tremendously variable and may be small at times and large at others depending on availability and purity. In 1986 'street level' samples of heroin in Edinburgh showed purities of up to 40% heroin, implying a well supplied market (see Fig. 2.2). The contaminant indicates the source to be probably Pakistan.

Fig. 2.2　*Analysis of illegal heroin – Edinburgh, June 1986*

1　The sample weighed 100 milligrammes.
2　The sample contained 38% diamorphine.
3　The sample contained 5% methaqualone.
　Cost (Black Market) £10.00

In addition to active drug ingredients which may, along with the heroin content, account for 50% of the powder taken, there are non-active substances present. These are also variable and the main requirements are that they will dissolve when prepared for injection. Frequently such contaminants do not dissolve but are suspended in the solution causing, presumably minor, tissue damage when injected. Talcum powder is often used and is contained in some tablets which are injected.

Examples of other more damaging powders, such as brick dust and detergents, are unusual and represent disorganization in the local supply system. More common is the use of dextrose or glucose, which readily dissolves in small quantities of water and has no damaging effects itself. The preparations used to mix substances and the methods employed are, however, not sterile and the possibility of injecting septic material is high.

The presence of unknown adulterants in illicit heroin is a source of concern for drug users and those involved with treatment. Although overdosage is commonly attributed to variation in purity or loss of tolerance, little is known about the truth of this assumption and several facts do not support this simple explanation. Overdosage, fatal and near fatal, often seems to occur in experienced users with no apparent loss of tolerance. Similarly many people die after injecting quantities of material which other people survive without noticeable effects.

A frequently observed explanation is the presence of other drugs in the body. Heroin users may well indulge in other drugs and the combined effects are much more likely to be fatal. Thus alcohol, paracetamol, barbiturates, dextropropoxyphene, methadone and others may account for such sudden deaths.

Modes of Administration

Many drugs or substances not commonly regarded as drugs are taken by all of us throughout our lifetime, and the mode of use is often felt to reflect the power of a compound to affect the body. Dependence, however, is known to result from inhalation, ingestion (eating) or injection of a substance such as heroin. The effects of the drug vary as does the quantity required, depending on the route of administration.

Tobacco and cannabis, if smoked, are absorbed into the bloodstream through the lungs and with increasing frequency this route is being used to take heroin. Heating the drug directly on a piece of tin foil causes it to vaporize and allows the fumes to be inhaled. This is known as 'chasing the dragon' or 'Chinesing' and is an increasingly popular way of using the drug. Similarly cocaine is used by many sectors of society as a stimulant when inhaled, or snorted, and absorbed through the nasal mucous membranes. Heroin can also be used in this way. 'Free-base' cocaine, a preparation which can be smoked, is increasingly available in parts of North America and Europe.

The traditional use in the East has always been by inhalation or by eating opium or its derivatives. In the West, and increasingly in parts of the East, the preferred traditional route is by hypodermic injection. Hypodermic as a term simply means beneath the skin and can include introduction of the drug into a vein or other blood vessel, into muscle tissue or subcutaneous fat just below the surface of the skin. All these techniques have their dangers and all can introduce toxins, chemicals or infections. Injection is preferred by many because of the comparatively small amount of drug required, making it the most cost effective use. It also provides the unique 'rush', a pleasurable sensation associated with a sudden introduction of heroin to the brain. This reaction is also sought by those injecting cocaine, when the lasting effect is more transitory and therefore administration more frequent.

Other types of injection of the drug are often used when available veins have been damaged or blocked and are not usable. In an attempt to introduce the drug into a vein, those in the lower limbs may also be tried and use of the femoral vein in the groin may be a feature of long use when the arm veins and small veins in the legs have been damaged extensively. This large vein runs close to the artery and nerve supply to the leg and therefore its use has particular dangers. It is, however, often preferred by people injecting irritant drugs such as dipipanone (Diconal), as it carries the drug into the main bloodstream more quickly.

Injection into skin, fat or muscle causes problems at these sites and if injection technique is poor, then abscess or local infection is common. The idea that the drug is less addictive if administered in this way is, of course, erroneous.

The mode of administration chosen for individual use has important effects on the health of that person. Moreover, the prevalence of injection of heroin worldwide has extremely important consequences for the health and economy of society as a whole. Physically damaging techniques result in medical problems and this clearly costs increasing amounts in medical time, equipment and expertise. The estimated 100,000 carriers of the AIDS virus in New York in 1986 represent about half of those using injectable heroin and/or cocaine, the total number of users being 200,000. In some parts of Europe (Spain, Italy, Scotland) similar percentages of intravenous drug users have been found to be affected. These infected individuals may become ill but are unlikely to die quickly. Even if remaining well, they may remain active and infective for many years. Either way, once established in a community, the virus will spread and people at risk will be those injecting drugs and those who are sexually active.

Patterns of Use

The type of drug used, those using the drug and how it is used, vary enormously throughout the world. They do, however, depend very much on what is available for consumption in any particular area or country and the establishment of a culture or subculture which in a way regulates its use and establishes local rules or moral values for what is and is not done. For a drug like cocaine therefore, there are widely differing rules about its use and these appear to be related to availability first and social position second. In common with most substances, if it is available then it will be used, at least by some members of society. Those who also use heroin by injection seem happy to inject cocaine as an alternative or as a substitute. A combination of both drugs used together is often taken when and where available. Cocaine, a stimulant drug and heroin, a depressant drug, have some opposing actions. In the more educated echelons of society, the drug is snorted or inhaled rather than injected and this is common in large North American and European cities. Availability very much determines the frequency of use and for obvious practical as well as historical reasons, it is currently more in use in the USA than Europe.

Heroin, similarly, has enjoyed an increasing availability bonanza in Europe over the last decade, and this has caused widespread use in areas previously devoid of the substance. Despite this, the patterns of heroin consumption have been different. Inhalation, traditionally more common in the East, has given rise to large numbers of heroin users over the years, but in such capitals as Bangkok the use of needles and syringes is widespread. The traditional use of these modern inventions in European capitals has, in recent years, been modified by an increasing number of those preferring to 'chase the dragon' in the Eastern way. Local differences persist in the use of heroin and other substances, legal and illegal, and a greater understanding of these variations may lead eventually to explanations as to why problems are encountered with heroin in different groups.

Conclusion

Heroin is undoubtedly a potentially very dangerous drug and the cause of much unhappiness and destruction to individuals and to society. To under-stand why it can be used to such benefit medically and yet to such destruction in an uncontrolled way, is complicated and depends on the person taking it and how it is taken. The vague notion of 'addiction' is not adequate to explain its use, and persistent use, in the face of overwhelming reasons for not continuing with this damaging behaviour. The many problems in pinning down the terms 'addiction' or 'addict' show up the complexity of the behaviour and the variation of individuals involved.

As in other areas of behavioural abnormality, boundaries between normal and abnormal are being broken down. Individuals can no longer be satisfactorily categorized as neurotic or stable. People have aspects or elements of both in their personalities. In the same way they have some elements which may be considered to be 'addictive' traits in their make-up and, under the appropriate conditions, exhibit those features which are present in illicit drug users.

Extensive physical or psychological manifestations of dependent behaviour may occur for reasons unrelated to the drug itself but to a combination of social circumstances, personal problems and drug use. The next chapter will confront some of the social problems and consequences which highlight drug dependence. In addition it attempts to elaborate why it is important to consider heroin use as a part of a complex group of personal problems rather than the cause of those problems. The ability to see through the web of popular myths to the individual person is the fundamental requirement for intervention or treatment.

3   Social Consequences

Although opiate dependence, or at least opiate use, has existed for a long time, the awareness of its presence has never before been so intense. The European picture has undoubtedly changed rapidly in the last decade, during which time the inexorable increase in numbers using heroin in North America has continued. But it is not just the numbers of individuals using heroin that has caught the public attention.

Interest in heroin has emerged from the traditional centres of London, Berlin, Amsterdam and New York to become a significant reality for most cities over half a million population and from there has gradually disseminated itself into the smallest towns and villages. No longer is heroin use a remote activity confined to the great cities. Even at a distance from a main centre of population and commerce, the drug is being used by an increasing number of young people. From the previous situation of regarding it as somebody else's problem, it now becomes an issue which has to be taken seriously and there can be few citizens without a point of view on the subject of heroin use and misuse. Many of these attitudes are formulated as a result of information supplied by the media and press, and the association of drug users with the AIDS virus has further increased attention.

This chapter will identify some of the problem areas resulting from heroin use. Without attempting to solve intractable areas of difficulty it will look at a few facts and attitudes towards them.

Estimates of Numbers of Heroin Users

The attempt to identify absolute numbers of people using any drug is bound to be wildly inaccurate and of comparatively little practical use other than perhaps in planning services. It has the significant disadvantage of supplying information that may be potentially damaging. The information that there may be 100,000 individuals in the UK who have tried heroin is of little value if one has no idea about the nature or extent of their involvement. Of the applicants to a Philadelphia methadone treatment programme in 1974, only

45% were found to be actually dependent on heroin. Similar estimates of the percentages actually dependent on the drug have been suggested from other sources. Indeed some national research in the US has suggested that only 10% of heroin users may be physically dependent on the drug.

It is apparent that numbers of those using the drug are increasing in many countries. The numbers of habitual users of heroin in the USA in the late 1960s were variously estimated at 15,000 to 300,000, the later figure being 0.1% of the population. In 1979 the National Institute on Drug Abuse (NIDA) estimated that there were between 387,000 and 453,000 heroin users in the USA. Hunt and Chambers estimated in 1974 that 3–4 million US citizens had used heroin although only 10% were dependent upon it. In New York City in 1980 the estimate was that about 200,000 individuals used heroin on some basis.

Official figures in the UK are considerably lower and from a few hundred in the 1960s, the Home Office Statistical Bulletin in 1984 recorded 5,415 new heroin users and 1,995 former addicts receiving treatment, a total of 7,410. Official sources estimate that this should be multiplied by at least 5 to give a realistic assessment of the actual prevalence of heroin users in the country, 37,050 total. Other sources would increase this considerably and many sources consider that in 1986 there were 100,000 heroin users in the UK.

In European countries accurate estimates are in short supply, but in Amsterdam alone it is thought that there are at least 6,000 individuals using heroin, although this may be inflated by incoming visitors from France and West Germany where policies on control and treatment are less liberal.

Aetiologics

The inevitable question of why the drug problem has emerged with such force and speed in the UK is not an easy one to answer. The reason for this is that, as in most aspects of social behaviour, a number of factors must be considered. The major factors in this particular aspect of social behaviour are probably simple and apparently coincidental. However, the fact that several areas of Europe have seen a similar increase in the problem suggests that there is one single factor operating. Availability of drugs is clearly a prerequisite for the emergence of a group of users. Well documented evidence of drug trafficking on an unprecedented scale has identified new sources of heroin in Pakistan, Afghanistan and Iran. These appear to have taken over from the traditional centres of production in the Golden Triangle of Burma and Thailand. The targeting of Western Europe as a market place for these production areas has been staggeringly successful and one wonders why it took so long to achieve this enormous breakthrough by those involved with organized crime.

Probably, therefore, the single most important causal factor of heroin misuse is that it is there now and was not there before. This single factor is also seen to operate in other fields of drug misuse and much pressure by the health lobby has drawn attention to the increased per capita consumption of alcohol associated with the declining real cost of alcoholic drinks (Royal College of Psychiatrists 1981). This may be an important factor in the increasing number of problem drinkers today.

Availability of heroin is only comparative and obviously legal constraints and social convention make it inaccessible to the majority of the population. It is not therefore the only factor accounting for the increased popularity of heroin. Social conditions and unemployment give rise to many personal difficulties and the disproportionate distribution of heroin users in low socio-economic groups adds further weight to this. The hopelessness and despair associated with poor or non-existent prospects have been shown to be a powerful stimulus to criminality and alcohol abuse, and the associated use of psychoactive drugs by those with diminishing hope for the future is, on the face of it, rather obvious.

Much has been said and written about the negative features of heroin use, the damage it can cause and the problems it leads to, but despite this, there are many new recruits every day. As a lifestyle it must therefore have some positive features, unless hopeless dependence is the only driving force. As discussed previously, such dependence is a variable entity and, indeed, for many drug users is not even a reality. Involvement with heroin means involvement with a peer group and with a lifestyle peculiar to that group. In order to maintain an income that will provide two or three doses of heroin a day, money has to be earned in one way or another. The daily drug supply has to be secured and this, for many reasons, may be difficult. If no supply is available then alternatives need to be considered and this may or may not involve the medical profession or others with access to drugs. The average day of a heroin user, during a phase of drugtaking, is therefore a busy one and the high cost of the drug necessitates a daily supply of money. For an individual, the lifestyle of a drug user may fill the purpose of an occupation, a purposeful daily activity providing stimulation, industry and satisfaction. The user has status among peers which can be enhanced by behaviour or performance in the act of the street user. The user has the support of that part of society with which he has chosen to identify and, despite alienation from the larger community, the user's position has, at least in the short term, all the requirements for living. The idea that the status of a heroin user equates with that of someone in conventional employment is often ignored.

An understanding of such a lifestyle should not be difficult if one recognizes that heroin use itself provides for enjoyment, social contact, social status and employment, albeit illegal in many cases. All the negative features have to be weighed against these positive requirements which all people have. Unemployment has a low status in society and carries with it a lack of purposeful activity, an absence of a structure to life and an identification with a peer group with no particular redeeming feature. A low income may seem to preclude any glamour in life and the ability to cope with such a negative position in a positive way may separate those with initiative and personality. The choice of heroin use as an occupational substitute may not be as illogical or bizarre as it might seem to those with prospects for following a more conventional career.

One of the more popular causal theories advanced to account for heroin use is that of mental illness. That drug users are ill and, specifically, mentally unbalanced is a common view. This has prompted the establishment of psychiatric institutions as the main traditional centres for therapy. Undoubtedly, there is considerable evidence that socially maladjusted individuals, who might well be considered psychopathic, are well represented in any group of heroin users, as they are in groups misusing other drugs or in confrontation with the law in many ways. It is, however, equally true that most opiate users have no obvious psychiatric illness and often come from unremarkable backgrounds or from high-status families. The relationship between psychiatric illness and drug use is again unclear. The cause of both drug use and misuse is complex and confusing. Many factors combine to prompt and foster both use and misuse. These include the user's characteristics, environmental factors and the chemistry of the drug or drugs involved.

A final consideration in the list of possible causative factors may be expressed as social pressures, or the reaction to public pressures. This rather vague notion that an individual might be encouraged to use a drug by the society in which he or she lives is not a new or unique concept. The national awareness of the dangers of advertising cigarettes, and to a lesser extent alcohol, has arisen out of the belief that the association of glamour, excitement and attractive personalities such as film stars or sporting celebrities with these drugs is likely to encourage use. The negative messages of lung cancer or heart disease are presented in a form less likely to be noticed by someone looking for pleasure and excitement. The presentation of heroin may not be quite so overt but the awareness that many people use intoxicating drugs gives credibility to the concept that drugs are fun. The reality for many individuals is that drugs *are* fun and this is because they supply excitement, risks, challenge, companionship and, in a way, some glamour in what might otherwise be a dull existence.

Public Reaction

Politicians, press and a proportion of the public are unanimous in their condemnation of heroin use as the major, if not the greatest, social evil of our times. Interestingly, the view of successive British Government advisory committees that it was a medical and social problem rather than a criminal problem meant that, in this country, the public reaction was more restrained and less condemnatory than in the USA.

The events of the 1980s, however, have seen a complete turnabout in the policies of the British Government, despite the continued medico-sociological views of their advisors, to bring thinking and policy very much in line with American principles. Thus the declaration of war on drug traffickers and users by the Nixon administration in the early 1970s and the promotion of drug pushers to 'Public Enemy No. 1' have been reflected in high profile political posturing by the Thatcher Government of the early 1980s.

Within and behind the policies are a wide variety of motives and objectives and although the change of direction and consequent change of attitudes are results of an alarming and worrying situation, the wisdom and logic of this approach is questionable. Much political and press coverage has concentrated on the drug trade and drug traders as having responsibility for damage to property and persons. Others, however, see the problems arising out of drug use as a consequence rather than a cause, and recognize the underlying malaise in society caused by unemployment, bad social conditions, frustrations related to inequality and lack of opportunities. The drug user has been widely used as a scapegoat for many recent social and medical problems and the cost, based on the flimsiest data, has been calculated in enormous terms. Whether or not these social problems would have arisen in the absence of heroin, and blamed on some other factor, will never be clear and it is therefore a scapegoat that can be used without fear of contradiction. To quantify the social costs of heroin use is not possible, but to understand how and why most people react as they do is as important as a search for the elusive cure.

Another consequence of the recent high public profile of the heroin problem has been the separation between this drug and other drugs. From the confusion in the public minds of the 1960s, when a series of new drug problems with amphetamines, barbiturates, cocaine, cannabis, LSD and morphine became linked inextricably as the 'drug problem' and the effects and consequences were seen as identical, the present awareness of heroin as a different drug with different problems has perhaps gone to the opposite extreme. The anxiety about other drugs has waned and the recognition of the dangers of these, as well as legal drugs such as alcohol, tobacco and prescribed tranquillizers, has been put to one side. It seems that public and policy makers can only think about one drug at a time. This creates an anomalous situation where many real dangers are concealed by the furore created by the media over heroin. Interestingly, the drug scene in London in the late 1960s was virtually dependent on medical prescribing and a large component of the problem still revolves round prescribed drugs. A recent survey of death certificates for the UK demonstrated the dangers of drugs prescribed to treat heroin dependence. It may be that society's handling of this particular problem is causing damage rather than providing a solution.

Crime and Punishment

Most cultures have adopted a largely punitive approach to heroin use. Identification of drug users as criminals because of their use of an illegal substance, and their association with the illicit traders in that substance, has made them distinct from those dependent on, for example, alcohol or cigarettes. The further involvement in crime to finance the illegal activity increases the perception of the individual as a criminal rather than a victim.

Whether or not this is correct or fair, the status of heroin users as criminals first and people with problems second is continually reinforced by the courts, the law enforcement agencies and the media. The result is, for most of the public, an almost inevitable conclusion that this is a true representation not only of some drug users but of all those involved at whatever level. A further consequence is the establishment of this belief even amongst those using the drug, and the development of a status outside the bulk of society occupied by those initiated by virtue of their drug experiences. Heroin use therefore introduces an individual into a group of *cognoscenti* who further reinforce these beliefs. The fact that the group itself is, like most clubs, supportive of its initiates gives rise to one reason for difficulty in breaking away.

That criminal acts should be punished is an accepted part of all cultures. That drug related offences should carry a more severe sentence or stricture is less apparent logic unless it reflects the anxiety and distaste present in society about the use of heroin. At the present time in many countries a drug related offence is more likely to result in a prison sentence or, as in Malaysia, a death sentence, than a similar non drug related crime. Similarly, the possession of heroin, even in comparatively small quantities, can result in custodial sentencing of equal or more severity to that of manslaughter or even murder if intent to supply can be proved. This must clearly reflect the fear and loathing felt by society towards the drug and its users and sellers.

There is little evidence that imprisonment helps people to overcome drug problems. Accordingly, confining heroin users to prison may reflect fears that, since there is no cure, there is no other way to control these people.

'No-Cure-No-Remission' Hypothesis

Much of what has already been said about society's reaction to heroin use reflects the erroneous belief that once heroin has been tried then dependence is inevitable and that this is a permanent or fatal state. Despite this it has been known for a long time that in order to establish a physical or chemical dependence, the drug needs to be taken regularly over a period of time, probably at least several times per week over several weeks. After stopping the drug, the body will rapidly revert to a non-dependent state and any tolerance will be lost.

Most long-term follow-up studies of opiate users have demonstrated large numbers of people who stop, for whatever reasons, and remain apparently fit and healthy. This may happen at any stage of an individual's drug using 'career'.

In addition, many researchers have shown the fluctuating nature of drug problems of all sorts and this includes heroin. Use may be continuous or intermittent and variable. Remissions and relapses occur regularly, often in an individual pattern. A remission may continue over a long period of months or years and may indeed represent a cure or a long term abstinence. The concept of 'once an addict, always an addict' does not seem to be true for most problem drug users.

Pushers and Users

The definition of a 'pusher' or seller (dealer) of heroin may be anyone who resells even the smallest quantity of the drug. Convention, however, accepts that the pusher is someone who supplies the drug for personal profit, obviously at the expense of those who purchase and use it. This is generally regarded as a particularly unpleasant crime and hence the entitlement of the courts to impose a long and often parole-free custodial sentence. The boundary between user and dealer is often blurred. The majority of drug users at some time buy more than they require for immediate consumption or purely for personal use. Reselling of small quantities to friends is the norm and profits at this level are small. Most are users themselves and finance their own use in this way rather than indulging in other criminal activities. The pyramid of supply is a very broad based one, having a small number of non drug using agents at its apex and a large number of dependent users at its base. The comparatively easy access to the drug gained by being a supplier often leads to increased consumption by those in such a position, with resulting physical and psychological deterioration.

Supply at street level, therefore, is carried on by a large number of heroin users making small profits quickly dissipated on personal drugs use. The stereotype of pushers as those who hang around on street corners or outside schools and tempt newcomers to use drugs is equally fallacious and likely, if it did occur, to increase the chances of being arrested rather than increase profits.

The emotive term 'pusher' therefore is often used to emphasize a distinction between users and traders which sometimes simply does not exist. Levels of drugs possessed are often astonishingly low in those accused of dealing. However, the establishment in court of the individual's status as a supplier allows the imposition of a severe sentence.

Cocaine

Although widely abused internationally, this drug represents a smaller problem in Europe than it does in the USA. This is partly because of the comparatively restricted supply in Europe and partly because, at least by most of those using it, it is not injected. Used by inhalation in the affluent sections of society, it causes fewer immediate socially or personally damaging consequences. The financial implications often prove more devastating than those associated with the effects of the drug. In the USA, however, its greater availability to those who also use heroin gives rise to widespread intravenous use. Being a short-acting drug it is often administered at regular intervals throughout the day and night. One clear consequence of 20 or more injections per day is the increased danger of introduction of infected material.

Usually presented in a white powder form, the free-base preparation of cocaine is currently used in a similar way to the resin of cannabis, in combination with tobacco.

Purity of Heroin and Quantities Used

Unfortunately, information on purity and therefore quantities used by individuals in each 'shot', or on a daily basis, is dependent on information from police laboratories and accounts of illegal and therefore clandestine activities. Purity of drugs seized by police depends largely on the point in the distribution chain at which the drug has been intercepted. Thus seizures of less than one kilogram have already been adulterated and from then on down may well be adulterated or 'cut' with contaminants at every stage in the distribution network. This is a haphazard and irregular mechanism the lower down the system goes and therefore quantities are variable. At the bottom, or final distribution point before consumption, the purity may vary from 40% down, usually lower than 30%. Recent UK seizures of 15–20% purity therefore mean that there are 150–200 mg of pure heroin in a gram of adulterated heroin on the streets. This may cost a variable amount, depending on local supplies at the time, and the estimated intake of pure heroin in one New York study was 80 mg/day or a range of 30–150 mg. As purities drop due to (usually temporary) interruption of supply, intake is reduced or cash outlay increased.

The variability of intake and the intermittent nature of heroin use are vital features in our understanding of the patterns of drug abuse at the present time and the realization that many users use very variable amounts has important implications for treatment and management.

Age and Sex of Heroin Users

Having made passing reference to some personal characteristics of heroin users, it is useful to try to identify further features of the current users, at least to note any changes over successive decades. The predominance of heroin taking in the lower social class, with a notable but comparatively small number in the socially elite, represents something of a change from the middle class backgrounds of many of those using heroin in the 1960s. The establishment of maintenance methadone as a treatment in the early seventies led to an ongoing cohort of heroin users dependent on methadone who are now in their early to mid 30s. Despite this, in the UK national statistics demonstrate a progressive fall in the average age of those reported to be using heroin. The number under 21 years old has increased since 1980, since which time the proportion has gone from 13% in 1979 to 22% in 1984. Remembering the presence of the cohort from the previous wave of heroin use and misuse, this means that the majority involved in the statistics now are in the lower age group, probably under 21 years.

Interestingly, the increased representation of women amongst drug users is reflected in many studies as well as official figures, which show about 30% of heroin users to be female. In the sixties and early seventies, women represented 20–25% of users of heroin.

The importance of these changes in age and sex of drug users has various implications. The increased number of women indicates the likelihood of children born to drug users being potentially infected with the AIDS and hepatitis B viruses and the decreasing age has marked implications for educational establishments as well as family situations. It has been suggested (Bucknall & Robertson 1975) that employment of family bonds and institutional connections may be one positive way to influence a favourable outcome.

Registration with Home Office Drugs Branch (UK)

There is a legal requirement for any doctor to notify to the Home Office the name of an individual using heroin, cocaine or dipipanone within seven days of becoming aware of the fact. For many years the bulk of these notifications came from doctors working in drug dependency clinics. These are usually psychiatrists. In recent years, however, the percentage of cases notified from these centres has dropped progressively and the numbers being notified by general practitioners and prison medical officers has risen. The average age

Table 3.1 *Narcotic drug addicts notified to the Home Office during the year, numbers no longer recorded as addicts and number recorded at 31 December*

	Number of persons										
	1974	1975	1976	1977	1978	1979	1980	1981	1982	1983	1984
Addicts recorded as receiving notifiable drugs at 1 January	1,816	1,967	1,949	1,874	2,016	2,402	2,666	2,846	3,844	4,371	5,079
Persons notified during the year as addicts by medical practitioners:											
New addicts	870	922	984	1,109	1,347	1,597	1,600	2,248	2,793	4,186	5,415
Former addicts	566	536	541	622	753	788	841	1,063	1,325	1,678	1,995
Total notified during the year	1,436	1,458	1,525	1,731	2,100	2,385	2,441	3,311	4,118	5,864	7,410
Persons no longer recorded as addicts at 31 December:											
Removed by reason of death	77	68	63	40	60	49	73	46	49	80	86
Admitted to penal or other institution	388	484	513	442	484	553	429	546	607	782	1,308
No longer recorded as receiving notifiable drugs	820	924	1,024	1,107	1,170	1,519	1,759	1,721	2,935	4,294	5,226
Total no longer recorded	1,285	1,476	1,600	1,589	1,714	2,121	2,261	2,313	3,591	5,156	6,620
Addicts recorded as receiving notifiable drugs at 31 December	1,967	1,949	1,874	2,016	2,402	2,666	2,846	3,844	4,371	5,079	5,869

of those notified from general practice has significantly fallen. This swing towards a younger group and away from the traditional treatment centres has several important consequences for those planning treatment and research strategies; these will be discussed later. The fact, however, that first awareness of a person using heroin is now largely in the community or in prison reflects the changing pattern of those involved with the drug scene. The purpose of the Home Office register is primarily one of statistical use to provide information on the size and nature of the problem in the UK. In particular it is used to indicate trends. In addition, it provides a facility of reference for medical personnel to identify the status of a patient as a drug user.

Establishment of a name on the Home Office register does not entitle that individual to any special treatment or therapy. In years past it was generally the case that the presence of an individual's name on the register implied that that person was attending a drug dependence clinic and therefore likely to be receiving a supply of prescribed drugs. Very few people attending such a clinic are prescribed heroin itself. Larger numbers receive a substitute opiate such as methadone. Today not only are clinics prescribing less, but most heroin users are notified by their own general practitioners or prison medical officers. The act of being registered therefore conveys no special status or privileges but allows only for official recognition of the changing patterns of use of these drugs.

Controlled Drugs

For the purpose of legal control of drugs considered to be dangerous, most Western countries and some others, the USSR for example, have a system of limiting the supply and availability to the medical profession and general public. In the nineteenth century, many opium and morphine containing compounds were freely available to the public in Europe and North America. Often present in large quantities in patent remedies, these resulted in considerable numbers of individuals being addicted. (In 1895 it was estimated that 2–4% of the American population were dependent on morphine.)

A series of statutes in both the UK and the USA established a light control over the legal supply and, in the USA, the decision to ban heroin even for medical purposes made it available only from illicit sources. The Harrison Act in 1914 in the USA was the first piece of legislation in that country to establish control over narcotic supply. This paved the way for the development of the criminal view of heroin or narcotic use. This was distinct from the British view, at that time and later, of the medical nature of drug dependence.

The 'British system' of prescribing heroin to dependants resulted from the reports of the Rolleston Committee in 1926 and the Brain Committee elaborated this by establishing drug treatment clinics throughout the country. These opened in 1967, enjoying a brief period of success first with heroin substitution therapy, then with injectable methadone and finally with oral equivalents. The clinic system has, in recent years, fallen into some disarray partly from inadequate support in terms of personnel and lack of confidence in this approach, and partly from overwhelming numbers of cases coming forward for treatment.

Substitution or Drug Free Therapy

This will be fully discussed at a later stage in the book but the social consequences of this dilemma remain of singular importance and therefore will be briefly mentioned here. Many times in the twentieth century history of drug problems, successive political or medical establishments have put forward opposing theories. Heroin, first synthesized in 1893, was not only available as a cough cure without prescription but was claimed to be a useful treatment for morphine dependence. The invention of methadone in Germany in 1941, as a useful drug in the management of those dependent upon heroin, was a similar example of the rather hopeful philosophy that substitution of a less noxious drug might lead to complete abstinence at a later stage. The establishment of increasing numbers of heroin users on substitutes, such as methadone in the 1960s and 1970s, has led to public anxiety about the cost of running such programmes as well as anxieties about their efficacy as a means of curing drug use. Poorly run programmes have been shown to have enormous problems, and efficient programmes integrated with psychosocial therapies and re-establishment of normal lifestyles are enormously expensive.

In the USA, the response to increasing numbers of heroin users has been to establish more places on maintenance programmes prescribing methadone substitution therapy. The unlimited numbers of individuals in some states, however, have exhausted these capabilities and the current situation is one of many ageing drug users attending maintenance clinics and many younger heroin or polydrug users rejecting or being rejected by this type of therapy. The 1960s saw a similar exhaustion of the smaller provision of clinic places in the UK, leading to a population of younger drug users throughout the country largely unaware of methadone substitution as a course of therapy. The observation of this group over a period of years may give critical information about the natural history of addiction in a group receiving minimal or no therapy. Other Scandinavian and European countries have adopted a similar rather aloof approach to the present epidemic of heroin use.

The Dutch experience of increasing numbers of heroin users in the years leading up to the present decade has been met in a variety of ways. A more liberal approach to heroin use, and indeed to other drug problems, has led to much international criticism and political pressure, especially from neigh-bouring countries. The existence of a union representing the users or 'Junkiebond' is a unique way of forging a link between the establishment and the drug users. This allows for the understanding of problems experienced by drug users and the provision of needles and syringes, as well as mobile distribution points of methadone on a daily basis. The mobility gives a regular contact point without the planning difficulties of allocating a building for the drug users. These measures are an attempt to normalize the lifestyles of drug users as well as reduce the risks associated with heroin taking. This initiative has had variable results. Of particular importance will be the effect on the spread of the AIDS virus.

Clearly there is little international consensus on the best way to manage the availability and control of heroin or synthetic opiates. Even if agreement were likely, it seems to be a situation controlled by numbers. Whatever system is initiated, resources are rapidly exhausted and the more liberal the system the more rapidly provision is used up. One thing is certain, the days of devising a law to control opiate use are gone. Moreover, the days of identifying absolute numbers using illicit drugs are gone and with them any hope of offering or delivering therapy to everyone with a 'drug related problem'. Perhaps this has one useful spin-off and that is an urgent requirement to re-examine the attitudes prevalent in society towards drug use; such as the hypocrisy of designating one drug as legal and therefore 'good' and 'safe' and another illegal and therefore 'bad' and 'dangerous', and the assumption that heroin users are a uniform group of deviants or criminals.

AIDS Virus Infection

Deliberately left to the ultimate part of the chapter on social consequences is the subject of the Acquired Immune Deficiency Syndrome. If heroin dependence was a social phenomenon in the 1950s, a medical problem in the 1960s and a political one in the 1970s, in the 1980s it has been designated a criminal problem. The undoubted place of many heroin users in the 1990s will be firstly in the realms of ethical considerations and secondly in the wards of infectious diseases hospitals.

Despite the fact that the largest proportion do not, and may not, become infected with the virus causing AIDS, anyone injecting any drug, not only heroin, beneath the skin runs a risk of exposure.

The established nature of the infection in drug users in many European and North American cities means that it is unlikely to go away whatever measures are taken now and whatever policies or laws are enacted. The infection is here to stay and will undoubtedly exert some influence on drug use and drug users.

The international debate, already well underway, on the best methods of preventing spread of the virus has to contend with many thorny ethical and practical difficulties. In a city like Amsterdam, with a history of a medical approach to heroin related problems, it is comparatively easy to implement such measures as the controlled distribution of sterile needles and syringes. In the UK, however, with its recent shift to the criminal or control view of drug problems, and in the USA with its policy toward heroin abuse monopolized by those agencies enforcing the law, this issue comes at a particularly difficult stage, not just for political reasons.

At no time in the past have drug users been such an isolated group, so distanced from any agency which might be capable of intervention. The AIDS virus has been characterized as a silent epidemic as it spreads invisibly through populations of sexually active men. The long delay from infection to onset of illness means that prevention requires long advanced anticipation. Even more silent is its spread in a risk group outside the law and outside society.

4   Patterns of Drug Use

Many factors contribute to the type of drug misuse which is adopted by an individual and there are as many variations in this as there are individuals. It is important, however, to have an understanding of the particular pattern present at any one time, in any one individual. Many types of substances are used and misused, often at the same time. Frequency of drug administration varies with time, a drug taker using large quantities at one phase in life and comparatively small quantities at others. Different substances have varied effects, physically and psychologically, and different modes of administration have important consequences. Some drugs, such as tobacco and alcohol, are legal and therefore do not lead to the crime and violence associated with illegal drugs. They also have the advantage of being prepared under sterile conditions and, being uncontaminated, the serious problems of infections and toxins do not arise. Their toxic effects are from the drugs themselves. They do, however, have the serious disadvantage that they are not perceived as dangerous by the drug user and therefore, being readily available, are often used indiscriminately. They are, of course, extremely dangerous drugs themselves.

Knowledge of the pattern of use and the types of substances being used is therefore a prerequisite for understanding the effects on an individual. Awareness that both of these factors change with time and availability of the substance leads on to an understanding of how treatment may vary from person to person, or from time to time or, indeed, from place to place. The everyday events in the lives of drug takers are examined below. This reveals the inconsistency and fluctuation which can be caused by many personal and environmental factors.

Polydrug Use

A rapid acceptance of this phenomenon over recent years has often distracted attention from the fact that many, if not most, regular drug users have a drug of personal preference. This is the one which is used most frequently, if not exclusively, by that person if it is available, like cigarettes or whisky in retail outlets. Not having the advantage of a regular or established supply, the illegal drug user often cannot get whichever drug he or she wishes. In this situation other drugs, often a wide variety, may be bought and taken. Many people use one or two drugs and will readily switch from one to another, using a third or fourth alternative only if absolutely necessary. Regional variation exists in the drugs available on the illicit market and this can be seen between countries or even between regions of one country. North America, for example, has a large and accessible supply of cocaine and this is used by a large part of the community. In the United Kingdom and Europe the supply is, for obvious geographical reasons, less uniform and at the time of writing remains comparatively restricted. Legally prescribed opiates likewise are readily available in some areas and comparatively restricted in others. The drug users in some cities in Europe have access to such analgesics as dipipanone (Diconal), dihydrocodeine (DF118) and latterly buprenorphine (Temgesic), all of which are abused orally and intravenously. Barbiturates, in great demand over many years on the black market, have, in some areas at least, become much harder to obtain than a decade ago. Local knowledge of these and other drugs therefore depends on two things; first, the illegal market which supports the importation of heroin and cocaine and, second, local or regional prescribing patterns and hence presence of drugs or tablets in retail and wholesale premises.

Use or misuse of drugs thus has noticeable regional and international variation and consequently the types of problems seen are often different. Users in New York injecting cocaine 10 or 20 times in one day will have a different pattern of problems from a London user inhaling heroin twice a week. The other drugs used, depending on local availability, will have some effect on the pattern of illegal drug use and this might be beneficial or, at times, detrimental. Whichever, it is clearly important to know what is available and therefore likely to be misused in a particular area. The inconsistency of the illegal market makes pressure on alternatives variable and there is good evidence that even those people receiving maintenance therapy in the form of pharmaceutical methadone, or other opiates, use a variety of illicit drugs during their therapy.

Drugs Abused

Although the opiate containing compounds, as well as cocaine and cannabis, are the main illegal drugs of misuse, there is no limit to the possible alternatives. Almost any pharmaceutical preparation may be taken, often in enormous doses, in an attempt to effect a psychoactive experience. Some will have that effect, often with a consequent danger from toxicity, others will have a damaging or lethal effect only, and many will be abandoned as useless.

To list the many drugs available to modern medicine, and therefore to misuse, is unnecessary. It is better to realize that there are large numbers of potential drugs of misuse. The single most important result of polydrug use and misuse is the possible interaction of a combination of substances. Recent information has suggested that many deaths in drug users are due to the toxic effects caused not by one drug but a combined damaging effect of two or more drugs taken at the same time or close together (Ghodse *et al.* 1985). The possible effect of alcohol and other legal drugs must also be considered. It has been shown that deaths are often due to a combination of an illegal drug and one or two legal ones, the latter usually including at least one opiate substance. The result is usually suppression of breathing caused by the combined opiate effect. Legal drugs therefore have a large and important part in the accidental death of drug users.

It must be of some concern to medical staff who seek to help drug users by legally prescribing supplies of opiates that these may be responsible for some deaths in this group. In addition to the opiates issued on prescription, there is the constant supply of other pharmaceutical preparations which leak onto the black market. Benzodiazepines and barbiturates, tricyclic antidepressants and sedatives all have a potentially lethal effect on their own but this increases in combination with an illegal drug such as heroin. Alcohol presents another hazard and potential pitfall for the unwary drug taker. Excessive alcohol consumption regularly accounts for long term physical damage in the form of coronary heart disease, cirrhosis, brain damage or blood vessel occlusion. It also can be of immediate danger, especially to those unaccustomed to large quantities or those taking it in combination with other substances. Thus its intoxicating properties may well potentiate the sedative and narcotic effects of opiates even to the extent of respiratory depression and death. Alone or in combination, it accounts for deaths due to accidents, overdosage and asphyxiation, deaths from hypothermia when exposure to excessive cold is unnoticed, and other causes.

Proprietary preparations are still available which contain active ingredients which may be misused. Cough suppressant mixtures containing codeine are perhaps those most often misused by those who are aware of the toxic effects. Small amounts (100–300 ml) of some of these preparations may contain the equivalent amount of opiate to an illegal dose of heroin.

Polydrug use is therefore of great importance. There are implications for those mixing different preparations and there are important considerations for those issuing prescriptions which may be abused directly or 'leak' into the illicit market. Price and availability have much to do with the pattern of drug use in a particular place at a particular time. Although the underground organizations which distribute the supplies of heroin, cocaine and cannabis to the West are responsible for that end of the market, the problems of London in the 1960s, Stockholm in the 1970s and perhaps many more cities in the 1980s, are a direct consequence of the inadvised but legal provision of barbiturates, amphetamines, benzodiazepines and alternative substances.

Patterns of Administration

The patterns of use of a substance often depend on availability to the consumer. Thus presence of readily available cocaine in a variety of forms in many parts of North America means that it is widely used by differing sections of the population. Within that population there is also a variety of patterns of use, the affluent generally using it by inhalation in a more controlled and less conspicuous way than the more chaotic polydrug misuser who may inject it several times a day, alone or in combination with other drugs. This gives rise to different manifestations of drug associated behaviour in these two groups. The former may have financial and domestic problems associated with a lifestyle dependent on drug use, whereas the latter might be expected to manifest the serious health consequences of drug injecting. Indeed, a recent study in New York showed a clear link between presence of the antibody to the AIDS virus and the intravenous use of cocaine (Schoenbaum 1986). Cocaine, however, is not available in the same unrestricted pattern in the UK or Europe and therefore presents few problems at the present time.

Other examples are many and the importance of the local pattern may be considered under these headings:

The drugs available locally.
The prevailing mode of use.
The prevailing infectious agents in the drug.
Using community and adulterants used.

The drugs available locally will depend both on legal and illegal sources and may vary over time. Supplies are irregular and dependent on police activity, thefts from pharmacies and the prescribing policies of local doctors. All these together give rise to a pool of available drugs at any one time.

Modes of use are subject to marked regional variations. Injection of opiates, cocaine, amphetamines or other drugs may be the usual pattern in some communities whereas others practice mainly oral or inhalational drugtaking. This may be partly local cultural activity and partly economic, less drug being required when taken by injection. This variation in behaviour may be considerable even between centres close to each other. It is of great importance as distinct policies may be required in the management of drug users in different centres.

The adulterants used and the presence or absence of infection in any group of drug users will influence the problems occurring in that group. A clean supply of injecting equipment and an uncontaminated supply of drugs might be expected to be associated with different problems. Thus bloodborne infections will spread rapidly throughout a group of drug users injecting with shared equipment. Similarly, a contaminated supply of drugs may account for a local outbreak of illness. The use of an impure or inappropriate substance will cause similar damage and the phlebitis and sepsis associated with injection of crushed tablets not prepared for intravenous use are often seen in outbreaks where such a supply has been made available.

Patterns of Drug Use Affecting Illness

Table 4.1 demonstrates a clear connection between a specific pattern of use and a damaging consequence, in this case the spread of bloodborne infectious disease. The viruses responsible for AIDS (HIV) and hepatitis B (HBV) are directly related to needle sharing activity. The AIDS virus is found to be less common in the Glasgow group and the main difference in behaviour between the two cities is the number of injections taken during the month of the research study. A pattern, in this case the needle and syringe sharing, accounts for the spread of these two diseases and the second factor, increased numbers of injections and increased numbers of partners, accounts for the presence of HIV in one group and not the other.

In a similar way the pattern of use of any drug by any method of administration will have a direct consequence on the problems arising out of its use. The drinking of the normal beverage ethyl alcohol contaminated with poisonous methyl alcohol (methylated spirits) might cause visual damage; the inhalation of solvents may cause lung damage in susceptible individuals; the injection of toxins or chemicals with a drug will cause damage to other tissues. The list is endless and indicates the need for awareness of local drugs and drugtaking practices rather than the acquisition of an encyclopaedic knowledge of drugs or possible side-effects.

Table 4.1   *Summary of intravenous drug abusers*

	Glasgow	*Edinburgh*
Number (male/female)	42 (26/16)	34 (24/10)
Mean age (and range)	21 (16–31)	22 (16–32)
Mean duration of heroin use (yr)	3.3 (0.25–7)	3.9 (1–11)
Seropositive (hepatitis markers)	14/36 (39%)	27/31 (87%)
Seropositive (HIV)	2/28 (7%)	17/32 (53%)
Mean heroin use (per week) (number of injections)	19	21

Abstinence and Relapse

The popular lay view of drug misuse maintains that those people taking heroin are likely to demonstrate one of two outcomes; they will die of the dangerous side-effects of the drug or its use, or they will continue to misuse the drug over a long period of time with resulting moral, physical and social deterioration. That opiate use can co-exist with an otherwise normal and useful lifestyle is not a fact that many people appreciate or find easy to cope with. This is mainly because the damaging effects are often far more evident than is controlled use. Heroin use may be damaging for many reasons, but it is sometimes used in a controlled way, as are other psychoactive drugs such as alcohol and cannabis.

Abundant evidence from both the USA and Europe indicates the presence of a group of heroin users who continue to work, or carry out useful and productive lives. More commonly, the changes which occur over a number of years in drug misusers seem to lead to an alteration in drugtaking behaviour. From a more sporadic and damaging style of drug misuse in early years, a more stable, less frequent and consequently less damaging type of heroin use develops. This appears to be related to the length of time over which drugs have been misused rather than the exact age of the individual. The existence of a group of stable drug misusers, and the likelihood of increasing stability in behaviour over a period of years, implies that the use of a drug like heroin might be compatible with leading a relatively normal life. The place of behaviour of this kind on the spectrum of drug use is discussed below, but some regular heroin users do not appear to become drug dependent.

Heroin use and misuse are not uniform conditions with an onset, a continuing phase and an end, but rather a series of ups and downs. Although this might appear to be stating the obvious, there has been little investigation of the patterns of heroin taking over a period of months or years. The recognition of spontaneous changes in drug users' behaviour and the further understanding that these are not related to therapy or prescriptions have led to an increased need for information about these changes. If drug use is reduced or ceases spontaneously, as a result of life events rather than professional intervention, is the latter necessary at all?

It is true that most, if not all, drug users have phases of abstinence or reduced drug use interspersed with heavy or damaging use. The comparative lengths of these intervals vary from person to person and may increase in length over a period of years. Longer periods spent off heroin are commoner in those using the drug for a long time and episodes of non-dependent use are frequent throughout. The significance of these changes is not often fully recognized by the drug user and the heavy user may not be prepared to admit that such a change has occurred in the past with minimal professional assistance. Nevertheless, phases of dependent use, non-dependent use and abstinence are an integral part of the lives of all heroin misusers and their importance is being increasingly recognized.

Occurring as they do sporadically and unpredictably, abstinent periods are in the same way followed by relapse and periods of dependent or non-dependent use. It seems logical therefore to direct intervention and therapy to the actual time of relapse, or the abstinent period, rather than to the using phase. This relapse prevention type of therapy is the basis of recent innovations which will be discussed later.

Non-dependent Drug Use

In Chapter 1 the nature of drug dependence was examined and also the difficulties in identifying one feature that might be said to be the diagnostic feature of dependence. That the main ingredient is a psychological craving and that physical dependence is a minor feature is long established, although not readily accepted by drug users or society. Consider first physical withdrawal. This is a cluster of symptoms, vague and non-specific in nature, which are attributed to the absence of the drug in the individual. Most of the work of agencies involved with drug users, and training of workers, initially centres round a series of educational lessons. The first of these exorcises the longstanding apocryphal stories of severe, protracted and devastating physical symptoms associated with withdrawal. Many books on the subject deal with graphic details of convulsions, delirium, confusion, profound abdominal pains, diarrhoea, spontaneous orgasms and many other severe symptoms. Whilst many of these undoubtedly happen in those suddenly withdrawn from enormous doses of heroin, many apply to barbiturate dependence and individuals who have built up tolerance to large doses of opiates. More usually, the drug user will experience these, or some of these, in a minor form. This might result from the comparatively small amounts used prior to abstinence or the type of drug and contaminant used most often. The amount of drug taken for withdrawal to be experienced on cessation of use varies from person to person, but below a certain level no physical withdrawal is felt. This level might be a few shots a week or less, but indicates what might be termed non-dependent use.

Psychological withdrawal is dose related to a lesser extent. That is, severe psychological withdrawal can occur after using only small quantities of the drug, whereas some people might not experience it though they have used large amounts of heroin. The psychological element in dependence, there-fore, may be viewed as less predictable, more difficult to deal with on a medical or social level and requiring some knowledge of personality, back-ground and present social and domestic conditions. The balance between physical and psychological dependence in any one individual is the key to understanding how to intervene and in what way to offer assistance. The way in which psychological dependence arises and the mechanisms causing it to continue are dealt with in Chapter 1.

Non-dependent use thus may occur at some stage in a heroin user's career. This may not be obvious to the user. He or she may be using small quantities of the drug because of supply problems, because of other social or domestic commitments or because of a real and intentional desire to reduce intake. There may co-exist a period of comparative psychological stability during which, for the same sort of reasons, less stress, anxiety or confusion is experienced. Progress can be made during this time in decision making, in self awareness and in gaining insight into personal behaviour. Episodes of physical and/or mental non-dependence are critical to understanding how best to intervene and if this sort of hiatus does exist, then identifying it and employing therapeutic resources could have a positive effect.

Periods of non-dependent use may be intermittent or, in the experience of many workers today, comparatively long lasting. The observation of long and stable periods of minimal heroin use is not new, but recognition is slow to affect the way in which therapeutic resources are deployed.

Non-dependent use is most commonly observed early in the lives of heroin users when, often at a young age, they have their first experience of the drug. At that time exposure may be intermittent for several reasons and lack of experience of the drug subculture means that, over a period of some months, only a few administrations of the drug are experienced. This is often the phase during which such individuals perceive their own drugtaking not as a problem but as a series of one-off events. The consequences of dependence and heavy use are not present and so anxiety is low and confidence about controlling drug use high. This early phase of non-dependent use may give rise to a more dependent phase, may result in long term damage from injection or, conversely, may lead to abstinence and no further drugtaking. This 'honeymoon period' may have an important influence on subsequent outcome. Even so, it is well known that during this time most see no professional worker or helper but derive most of their information about drugs from fellow drug takers or other friends.

The second phase of non-dependent use occurs later in the career of most of those taking heroin. Following the 'honeymoon period', which often continues for eight or nine months, there may be a long and sustained period of dependent use which may last several years if nothing happens during that time to affect it. This often coincides with changes in personal situation, a young adult living away from home for the first time being the most common example. The second phase of non-dependent use follows this prolonged and often damaging episode and is characterized by its transitory and sporadic nature. Over a period of months, or years, intermittent attempts at abstinence are evident and these may be very short indeed. A new pattern emerges over the next few months or years which clearly shows that, at least at times, problem free use has been present. These remissions and relapses follow an individual pattern in each drug taker and may be repetitive over a period of time.

Many opiate users mature out of drug use. This fact has important implications for the provision of services to help problem drug users and their families. More important still may be the increased understanding of what one might expect to see in any one individual over a period of time. Although any drug taker may abandon drug use at any time and may never restart, it is important for those offering help to understand that an equally likely pattern may be of remission and relapse. The evidence that these remissions may become frequent and more prolonged as time goes by provides for a new confidence that the long term outlook may not be as gloomy as often feared.

The increasing chances of death or disease during the periods of drug use must indicate a need for prevention of these consequences. The failure of previously tried methods to effect a change in drugtaking behaviour should sensibly give rise to recognition of more effective ways of intervention.

Abstinent Periods

All accounts of heroin use, personal or professional, describe periods of time spent taking no drugs. This is often in between episodes of heavy use and attention or interest tends to be drawn towards the description of this rather than the account of the drug-free time. That these times exist in the life of any heroin user is clear and not in dispute. What is needed now is a clearer idea of why these times off drugs occur and which factors cause relapse. Also, knowledge of the problems encountered and the successes and failures in daily living during the drug-free episodes is lacking. Without this information it is impossible to understand why any one person might relapse, or how this might best be prevented. Building on success is a more positive approach to any problem than attempting to patch up a crisis.

Conclusion

This chapter is intended to demonstrate two things. One is the variability in patterns of drug use and misuse and the many individual and personal factors which make each drug user a unique prospect for the counsellor or therapist. The second important concept is that of recreational or non-dependent use. This is not only poorly recognized by society but little understood by drug users themselves. Like all people, drug users are subject to propaganda, mythology and much of the received wisdom about drug use which is popularized by the media as well as the drug subculture itself. A drug user might find it difficult to believe that withdrawal may be achieved with minimal pain, or that he or she has indeed been 'cured' many times in the past, and therefore may have insurmountable psychological barriers to progress. Society may prefer to perpetuate many frightening myths rather than face the reality, which has enormous implications economically and for social change. For a politician to admit that marked social pressures foster heroin use might be politically dangerous. Even to accept that many heroin users are only dependent for short periods of time, and that current strategies for dealing with this are often counterproductive, is not likely to be well received. Society dares not accept psychological dependence but prefers to attribute the damage to physical causes.

The plastic nature of drug use as a behaviour pattern and the variations in individuals or groups within that pattern are there to be seen. Success in managing or coping with drug use depends very much on the acceptance of this.

5   Illness and Death

It is a curious conundrum that heroin, when used in controlled doses under sterile conditions, is a relatively non-toxic drug. There are many well documented cases of people using heroin, either intravenously or by inhalation, for many years with no evident ill effects. Most drug counsellors and clinicians are well aware that many drug users can appear perfectly normal, even at a time of comparatively heavy drug use, and that heroin use can be compatible with healthy appearance and longevity. In addition, those heroin users who have given up the habit, provided they have not contracted any disease during their drug use, may be expected to enjoy a more or less normal life span. This may not be true of people who abstain from excessive alcohol use or some of those who have used tobacco. Indeed these latter two drugs have a remarkable ability to damage specific organs in the body. Tobacco is toxic to lung tissue and heart blood vessels, and ethyl alcohol can cause irreversible damage to brain, liver, kidney, heart, gut and other tissues. Opiates, perhaps because they represent a molecule similar to naturally produced chemicals in the body, appear to cause no 'end organ' damage of this nature and problems arising out of use are mainly accounted for by contaminants, the administration of septic material along with the drug, the transmission of infected material from cross-contamination from another individual or by excessive overdosage. Removing all these dangers, which are obviously considerable, the use of opiate drugs even intravenously is surprisingly non-toxic. The psychological effects of the drug on behaviour account for the major harmful consequences associated with drug use.

Physical Damage

In order to illustrate the major medical complications of heroin misuse, a review was conducted of some of the reports appearing in medical and psychiatric journals in 1985. In the area of complications due to heroin abuse, 31 separate articles from many different European, American and other journals appeared that year. Of these, 22 were directly related to infective agents. In some of these reports, the authors considered the infection to have been introduced by the needle and syringe used to inject the drug. In others, such as episodes of pneumonia, it was felt that the infective agent had been active primarily because of the general ill health of the patient rather than because of its route of introduction. However, the majority of illnesses were clearly caused by contaminated injections. On some occasions this gave rise to specific tissue or organ damage, such as the fungal eye infections reported from Australia, America and Scotland, and the widespread skin boils and abscesses caused by the same organism. Generalized infections, such as toxoplasmosis and malaria, as well as brucellosis and tetanus, have been reported during this time.

Other conditions less clearly related to infection and therefore possibly caused by general effects of the drug on the body's immune response are noted in kidney and brain tissue. Disorders thought to be due to the effect of the drug on the brain, causing conditions such as depression, have also been reported.

The prevalence of infections in the list of complications (Table 5.1) shows this as the main source of medical problems in heroin users.

The additional observation that many of these problems appear to occur in clusters, or minor and localized outbreaks, deserves further consideration. These outbreaks are demonstrated by reports from centres far apart and having the same explanation. It may be that an initial observation by one worker gives rise to increased awareness in others, resulting in those

Table 5.1 *Medical disorders listed as 'Complications of Heroin Dependence' in Index Medicus (cumulative) in a single year (1985)*

Pulmonary candidiasis (fungal lung infection)
Bacterial endocarditis (heart valve infection)
Depression
Tetanus
Infected subclavian aneurysm (blood vessel infection)
Neuropathy (nerve damage)
Toxoplasmosis (infection)
Malaria
Pneumonia
Septic arthritis (joint infection)
Fungal endocarditis (fungal infection of heart)
Globus pallidus (brain) damage
Ischaemia of extremities
Splenic abscess
Brucellosis
Endophthalmitis (eye infection causing blindness)

individuals looking out for similar cases in their own population of drug users, or it may be that because of behaviour change, minor epidemics of complications do appear in different centres.

Physical harm, therefore, is a formidable subject and, in the area of heroin misuse, covers a wide range of conditions. The most prevalent ones are clear, however, and those unusual conditions which are rare will not be discussed further, except in general terms. The important complications can perhaps be most easily examined under some general headings:

Lifestyle and behaviour-related.
Infectious disease-related.
General health-related.
Overdose – fatal and non-fatal.
Epidemics of infection.
Future trends.

Lifestyle and Behaviour

That drug use and misuse exists in all strata of society appears to be generally accepted, and the use of heroin and cocaine is clearly included. Also generally recognized, at least by those involved with treatment, is that the most damaging effects of drug abuse arise when it is taken in an impure, adulterated or infected form. Someone who is able to afford a clean and pure supply from a source unlikely to add toxic contaminants is less likely to be affected by problems. In addition, the individual who understands the potential dangers and is able, either through position or influence, to obtain the necessary equipment or advice that will prevent problems, is in a position of comparative safety.

Damaging behaviour or lifestyles arise when these situations do not prevail and when, through additional factors, self-preservation is not considered. These factors may be the very reason for drug use in the first place and may therefore be seen as the real cause of the damage to health. In the same way as an individual will use a sharp knife to cut his throat, or a bottle of aspirin to commit suicide, heroin can be seen as the way of carrying out a damaging act. The treatment should be directed at the underlying conditions or causes. Many explanations of drug misuse have been advanced. It is widely conceded that drug use and misuse may be caused or influenced by a host of factors connected with personality, position and environment.

For whatever reason, some individuals are prepared to harm or neglect themselves. Perhaps the psychological effects of drug use lead to loss of interest in appearance, in social conventions, in simple vital acts such as ensuring an adequate diet. Weight loss is a common consequence of heroin misuse and this is largely due to dietary neglect. Failure to eat an adequate, varied range of food leads to general malaise or even nausea. Constipation is common due to a combination of poor nutrition and the effects of the drug on the bowel. This may lead to haemorrhoids and other painful conditions. Vitamin deficiency and skin disorders may further increase discomfort and a predisposition to infections may cause general ill health. Chest infections are common, perhaps due to concomitant cigarette smoking, and this may also account for the insomnia which is a commonplace complaint, especially during periods of withdrawal when cigarette consumption may increase dramatically. Large amounts of tea or coffee may also be taken increasing agitation or insomnia during episodes of decreased opiate use.

Many of these features in isolation might account for bodily discomfort, often of an extreme degree. In combination they are sufficient to make the strongest individuals feel sorry for themselves and often may account for a large part of the withdrawal syndrome.

Lifestyles may additionally be harmful to the drug user because of the associations that are bound to be made to obtain an illegal drug such as heroin. It is clear that the drug user is living in a violent, or potentially violent, world. The life is one of risk and confrontation with peers, criminals, police and society and therefore violent acts are commonplace. Trauma of a different nature may arise out of accidental injury whilst under the influence of a drug or through the neglect of personal safety standards.

Infectious Diseases

Although the most serious and damaging examples of infectious diseases must be those caused by intravenous drug use, many others such as chest infections occur in debilitated drug users. Sexually transmitted diseases occur, as they do in the general population, but may be more severe due to lack of resistance brought about by all the features discussed above. Repeated or severe venereal infections may give rise to infertility, especially in women.

Skin conditions caused by injections are common and usually result from failure to inject the substance completely into the vein. Leakage into the tissues around the vein gives rise to local irritation, especially when tablets containing talc have been used. Infection introduced in this way will cause abscesses at the site of inoculation or spreading infection, called cellulitis, from that point outwards. These infections may increase to the extent that they cause illnesses such as fever, sweats, rigors and even generalized infection with all the serious consequences that that implies. Most intravenous users of drugs experience repeated and comparatively minor problems of infection in veins in the arms or legs. This may give rise to blockage in the vein which may or may not recover. The long term injector therefore may exhaust the majority of veins in this way. Specific problems with obstruction of a vein may be observed in the drug user injecting dipipanone (Diconal) which is especially irritant. Cases are described where obstruction has occurred in a major vein remote from the site of injection and this may well be fatal.

Before the introduction of the AIDS virus into the drug using population, the major problems of infection, caused by injection of contaminated materials, were hepatitis B and bacterial endocarditis – or infection of the valves of the heart. The latter problem is perhaps less common although, for some unexplained reason, it occurred in many individuals using intravenous drugs in several centres during 1983–84. This was presumably due to an infected batch of heroin being distributed. Sporadic cases occur nevertheless and the disorder is caused by the colonization of the valves of the heart by a bacterium or, less commonly, another infectious agent. Like an infected focus elsewhere, this causes damage to the edges of the valves with consequent impairment of their vital functioning. Treated early and adequately, this infection may well be halted but, depending upon the damage already done, long term health may be impaired. In extreme and uncontrolled cases, small infected portions of tissue, or septic emboli, may dislodge from the valve and disseminate to brain or other tissue causing further damage. Destruction of a valve, or valves, may be so extensive that the heart cannot compensate and sudden death may occur. Intervention at the stage of extensive damage, by a surgical procedure to implant a new artificial valve, is often compromised by the drug user's continued use of heroin and the surgeon's reluctance to give the person priority over cases deemed to be more deserving.

Considering the injecting technique used by many drugtakers, it is surprising that more heart valves do not become infected. The reason for this is probably that there has to be some pre-existing valve damage in order for infection to lodge in that site. This damage may have been caused at an earlier stage in the patient's life by acute rheumatic fever or by congenital acquisition of an abnormal valve or valves.

Hepatitis

Hepatitis means inflammation of the liver and is therefore a general term. It can be caused by various means; drugs which have a directly toxic effect on liver cells, infections by parasites, bacteria or viruses, or unknown factors. When hepatitis is present in a young person using heroin intravenously it is probably caused by a virus, usually the hepatitis B virus. It must be remembered that, even in a drug user, there may be many causes of hepatitis and that the presence of antibodies to the hepatitis virus, or other signs of its presence in the blood, should be identified. Clinical symptoms of acute hepatitis such as nausea, malaise and abdominal pain or signs such as jaundice may be present. Many individuals claim never to have experienced symptoms and express surprise when blood samples indicate active or previous infection.

The absence of symptoms or signs of hepatitis does not therefore preclude the infection, nor does it mean that the individual will not develop some of the possible long-term consequences. In most groups of drug users studied at the present time, there is evidence of previous infection in a high proportion of samples taken. Levels may be as high as 85%, although many of these individuals deny exposure by needle sharing. This may represent failure to admit the facts or it may indicate the other main mode of transmission, which is sexual intercourse.

Acute infection may therefore be unrecognized or may be passed off as a minor series of symptoms and attributed to 'flu or some other illness. It may, however, present as acute illness of a severe nature resulting in nausea, vomiting, exhaustion, confusion and irritability, rarely leading to central nervous system symptoms, liver failure and death. The more common minor illnesses should not be disregarded as a passing irritation. Long-term consequences can be severe, a proportion of cases becoming chronic carriers and therefore representing an infective pool. These individuals may infect sexual partners and, if female, children born to them. A smaller proportion of these chronic carriers may develop active liver damage leading to cirrhosis and even cancer of the liver. It is important to recognize that although cancer of the liver is comparatively rare in the Western world, it is common in the Indian subcontinent and Africa. The fact that cancer of the liver is one of the top ten cancers in the world is attributed to the high prevalence of the virus in these countries. It may therefore be reasonable to expect that a small proportion of drug users will ultimately die of this disorder. Children born to recently infected mothers, or to mothers who are chronic carriers of active infection, are likely to become infected at birth. As the babies' immune system is immature, many may become chronic carriers and may therefore represent potential dangers to contemporaries as the child grows. Chronic liver damage of the types already discussed may occur in comparatively early life (Fig. 5.1, p. 70).

AIDS

The other blood and sexually transmitted disease which has many similarities, at least in who it appears to affect and why it affects them, is of course the HIV or AIDS virus. This appears to have been introduced into the drug using communities of New York and San Francisco during 1978 and somewhat later in the United Kingdom, appearing in Edinburgh in 1983 and Glasgow as late as March 1985. In a similar way to hepatitis, once the disease is established in a needle sharing and sexually active community, spread will increase rapidly as more and more individuals become infected. It is not difficult to see that even if only one person is infected then one might be

Fig. 5.1 *Types of liver damage resulting from hepatitis B*

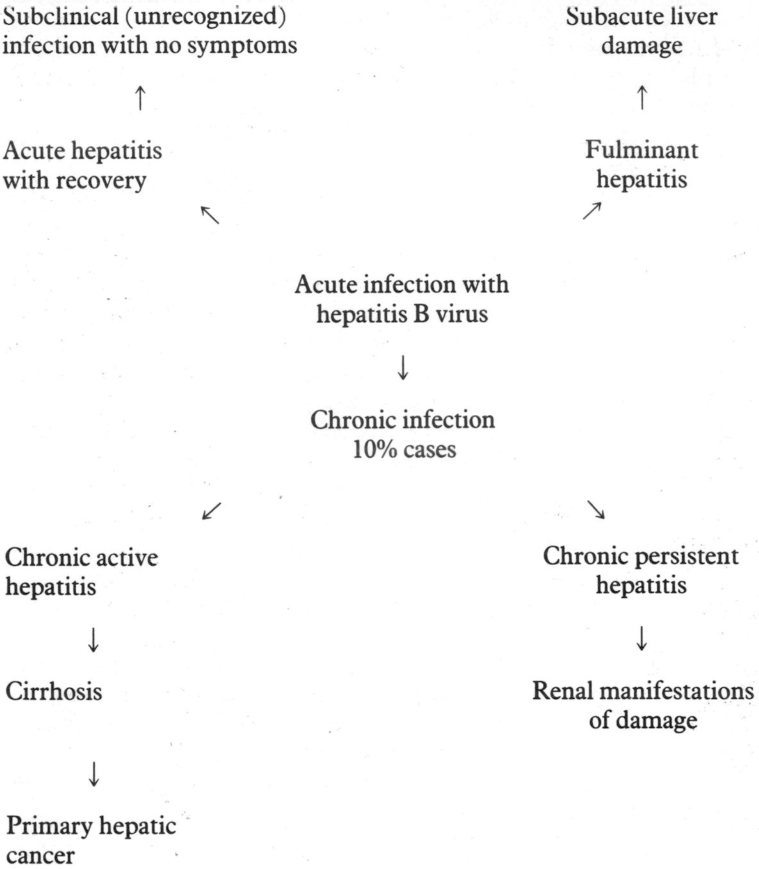

Subclinical (unrecognized)   Subacute liver
infection with no symptoms   damage

↑   ↑

Acute hepatitis   Fulminant
with recovery   hepatitis

↖   ↗

Acute infection with
hepatitis B virus

↓

Chronic infection
10% cases

↙   ↘

Chronic active   Chronic persistent
hepatitis   hepatitis

↓   ↓

Cirrhosis   Renal manifestations
                                                                 of damage

↓

Primary hepatic
cancer

unlucky enough to be sharing equipment with them. However, where many
are infected, each newcomer sharing needles is likely to be rapidly exposed to
infection. Why some centres have such a high percentage of infected people
remains unexplained and, at least in the USA, the time of arrival of the
infection in the community cannot be the only factor. HIV infection will be
discussed in full in Chapter 6.

General Health

General illness is not a necessary sequel to heroin abuse. Many individuals
maintain general health adequately even during periods of heavy drug use, in

the same way as those abusing alcohol may do. It is important to recognize possible areas of damage, particularly related to infectious disease, and at the same time to understand that heroin users are prone to the same illness as the rest of humanity under the same conditions.

In many accounts of medical observers dealing with heroin users, the need for attention is minimal in the absence of infectious disease. Frank neglect and problems which could be attributed to lifestyle are common and are not unique to those using drugs.

Separating out the damaging effects of heroin on the body from other causes is therefore difficult. A common example of this is the suppression of menstruation in some female opiate users. This is not a condition peculiar to heroin users, however, and can occur in a wide variety of totally different circumstances. The connection with stress, emotion or even weight loss is well known and these may co-exist with heroin use. The commonest cause of lack of a period in a young woman who is sexually active is, of course, pregnancy and this must be an early consideration. Pregnancy, however, is traditionally thought to be unlikely in those taking heroin and experiencing amenorrhoea (absence of menstruation). The assumption that amenorrhoea is associated with suppression of ovulation, and therefore with genuine infertility, may or may not be true. Certainly, in most women using large quantities of heroin, failure to conceive is the rule even in the absence of precautions such as the contraceptive pill. This state, however, seems to be reversible, periods returning when intake of the drug is reduced and normal fertility being re-established.

The common pattern of sporadic and intermittent use with episodes of often prolonged abstinence means that some women are more likely to menstruate and ovulate normally and hence have a good chance of becoming pregnant. Especially in the presence of the AIDS or hepatitis virus, or when exposure to these is possible, it is important that the dangers of pregnancy are understood and that infertility is not automatically assumed.

Overdose – Fatal and Non-fatal

Most people believe that overdosage of heroin is the usual cause of death in users of this drug. Commonly quoted figures put the annual death rate in groups of heroin users between 1% and 2% each year from all causes, and sudden death, assumed to be a fatal overdose of the drug, is usually quantified as the most important single cause. Overdose actually kills by depression of the central brain mechanism which activates respiration and this rapidly causes asphyxia and death. It is believed to occur when a user administers a dose of heroin which exceeds the personal limit of tolerance. Gossop (1982) reports that 'there seems to be no limit to the amount of opiate the body is capable of tolerating', although a dose of 200–300 mg or less may well be fatal to a non-tolerant user. Exceeding tolerance limits may occur in several ways: an experienced user may administer a dose of unusual purity (25–40% is not unusual in the UK at the present time), or become careless through desperation or other drug effects, or simply be unaware of the dangers.

Overdose may also occur following a loss of tolerance. If a person abstains from drug use for a reasonable time, tolerance to the drug will be lost and a previously acceptable dose may be enough to cause respiratory depression. Abrupt losses of tolerance are less easy to explain. Drug users have been known to overdose after taking quantities of heroin (from the same source) which were easily tolerated only hours before. One possible explanation for this has been proposed by Siegel et al. (1982). Their model of tolerance, based on Pavlovian conditioning, suggests that with each administration of the drug an association is made between the environment in which the drug taking occurs (the conditioned stimulus) and the generalized effects of the drug (the unconditioned stimulus). The environment therefore becomes a sufficient stimulus to induce an 'anticipatory response' which attenuates the effects of the drug, contributing to tolerance. Whether or not one believes this view, there is some evidence that drug taking in an unfamiliar environment is more likely to lead to problems.

Probably more important is the damage caused by a combination of drugs. The likelihood of overdosage increases when a heroin user takes other substances which may have depressant effect on the central nervous system. Ghodse et al. (1985) in their review of mortality of heroin users notified to the Home Office between 1967 and 1981, reported some interesting findings. These clearly indicated that the deaths of heroin users cannot be attributed solely to the drug itself. Only 74% of the deaths in this study were directly related to drugs, heroin being implicated in only 70% of these. It was concluded that many of the deaths were due to a combination of drugs being taken, the cumulative effect being the fatal factor. Many of the drugs implicated were those issued by medical prescription. A similar study of Home Office records by Bewley (1968) reported that accidental overdosage, sudden death following opiate administration, accounted for only 29% of deaths of heroin users. Suicides accounted for around 23%, the remainder being death by violence, septic conditions or natural causes.

A similar pattern was observed in a large American study carried out by Joe and Leishman (1982). Their follow-up of patients four years after treatment revealed that 28% of deaths were by violence, 17% natural causes, 44% drug related and 11% unknown.

The importance of other drugs as a factor in the aetiology of overdosage is therefore something to be considered. Of obvious importance are other opiates such as methadone, dihydrocodeine (DF118), buprenorphine (Temgesic) and codeine, some of which may be used in therapy. Important also are other commonly prescribed drugs which may be safe on their own but dangerous in combination or in excessive dosage. These include barbiturates, dextropropoxyphene and benzodiazepines. Reduction in their availability to the illicit market may have some effect on mortality due to overdosage.

Non-fatal overdosage is a little reported side-effect or complication which is seldom considered as such by drug users. However, anecdotal information gives an alarming incidence of episodes of loss of consciousness, prolonged intoxication and even lack of spontaneous breathing, when companions have had to stimulate breathing to prevent death.

Because of the illicit sources and the variable quantities of heroin available to those who rely on the black market, side-effects are common and transitory fevers and chills probably caused by bacteria viruses and toxins directly introduced into the bloodstream demonstrate how efficient the normal mechanisms are at dealing with some of these problems.

Epidemics of Infection

Minor or major epidemics are a feature of infectious illness and reflect a combination of factors present at any one time which enable transmission from host to host. The cramped, overcrowded conditions of Victorian Britain therefore allowed for epidemics of cholera, typhoid and tuberculosis, which largely disappeared when the conditions were altered by removing the source of infection or improving living conditions and reducing the direct spread. Those infections spread by aerosol or droplet affect communities in a different pattern from those spread by direct physical contact, and those spread by direct blood to blood contact will present a special risk for people that come into close contact with the blood of an infected person.

Thus intravenous drug use carries with it the possibility of dissemination of infectious agents and if conditions are right, then this may well occur in part or all of a community.

Epidemics of infection have been identified in drug users before and Bewley's observation of the rapid spread of hepatitis through the then small community of intravenous drug users in the UK in 1968 was a useful example of this. Previously, the frequency of this infection had been noted in the US amongst heroin users and those injecting amphetamines. Alter and Michael (1958) had reported an epidemic related to needle sharing between heroin users.

In this way, hepatitis B (serum hepatitis) is passed from drug user to drug user and from generation to generation of young people. Evidence suggests that large percentages of British heroin users in most centres have been infected at some time (Robertson 1986). Local epidemics appear to occur when conditions are right and this may be due to large numbers of newcomers joining an infected source or the change in behaviour due to alteration in availability of sterile equipment.

The AIDS or HIV virus has similarly been shown to spread rapidly through susceptible hosts, although the infectivity appears to be somewhat less than with the hepatitis B virus. Under some conditions the spread has been epidemic, as in New York or Edinburgh. Increasing evidence points to the conditions being right for spread in other European centres, notably in Italy, Spain and Yogoslavia, and not in others. This may relate to other factors such as sexual activity and practices, but it seems likely that the lack of sterile needles and syringes in some of these centres may account for the spread of the virus. Many pharmacists in London may be prepared to sell needles and syringes to drug users and this may account for the slow spread of the HIV infection in that city. Evans (1985) found that one chemist had sold 13,000 needles to known drug users.

Another infectious agent, long known as the source of a variety of disorders in drug users, is the yeast organism called *Candida albicans* which causes the disease called thrush. This has been shown to be responsible for odd episodes of abscess, endocarditis and generalized infection causing fever, chills, malaise and sickness. It does, however, occur as an epidemic, again under conditions suitable for its spread. This has been reported from several centres in the form of an eye infection (endophthalmitis), causing blindness if not treated early. Twenty three cases were recently reported from Glasgow and the underlying source was identified as lemon juice stored in a plastic bottle and repeatedly added to heroin to acidify the solution and facilitate dissolving. This particular minor epidemic is well understood, at least locally, and practices amongst drug users have been altered to avoid this. In a centre of similar drugtaking proportions, where citric acid crystals, available in chemist shops, are used to acidify the solution, these complications have not been recorded – again, a case of the conditions in Glasgow at that time allowing the spread of infectious agents.

Perhaps less well understood are episodes of heart valve infection (endocarditis) occurring in clusters, as reported from several North American and European cities. During the period 1982–1984 many cases were noticed in Manhattan, leading to the establishment of a research project to elucidate the source of infection and the mode of spread. As often happens with infectious diseases, the study found few new cases to research and conclusions were limited. A similar wave of cases occurred in the UK during the same period and subsequently seemed to vanish.

Clusters of overdoses have been observed in minor epidemics of drug related deaths. These may indicate contamination with toxins or infections or increased drug use. The increased death rate in the UK in the late 1960s, compared with that in New York, was thought to be due to one of two factors. Either there was a failure in New York to record correctly all deaths due to heroin use, or there was an over-estimate of the numbers of local drug users. Alternatively, there may have been an epidemic of drug related deaths in the UK at that time. Bucknall (1986) has demonstrated a reduced mortality in the early 1980s in a small study of intravenous drug takers.

Future Trends in Morbidity and Mortality

These are likely to be dominated by the AIDS virus, at least in those centres where the virus has become endemic. Mortality is likely to be considerably increased over the prevailing 1–2% per annum. A new era has arrived in which historical comparisons will become redundant. A new factor has entered the equation, weighting it more heavily than ever against the drug user sharing equipment. Morbidity in a similar way will be overtaken by this infection. A new range of complications, many of which we cannot imagine at the present time, will become evident in the next decade and infected survivors are likely to demonstrate a bewildering array of medical curiosities and conditions.

6 AIDS

What is AIDS?

First described in the USA in early 1981, this is an infectious disease caused by a virus now known as the human immunodeficiency virus (HIV). Previously this virus was known by French researchers as LAV (lymphadenopathy associated virus), and to American workers as HTLV III (human T cell lymphotrophic virus type III).

This virus causes a specific disease affecting the immune system by attacking the T cells which are that part of the defence mechanism which copes with infection. Similar viruses are known to exist in some species of African monkeys, but apparently they do not cause illness of the type seen in humans.

The resulting damage done to the immune system means that infections which normally are not harmful to the body become serious. Thus bacteria, viruses and fungi which are normally present in the body become dangerous to the tissues and organs. Patients suffering from AIDS therefore present with problems of infection, the causal agents being rather unusual and seen in other diseases or conditions where the immune system is inadequate. Thus the same sorts of infection may be seen in people with advanced malignant disease and those receiving drugs which suppress their immune system.

Common conditions associated with AIDS are therefore pneumonias, bowel infections causing fluid loss, poor nutrition and debilitating diarrhoea, invasion of organs or tissues by otherwise benign fungal growths and unusual tumours reflecting impaired resistance. Finally, the invasion of the central nervous system by the virus or by other organisms may result in signs of brain disease such as confusion, delirium or dementia.

The AIDS virus causes damage in an indirect way by destroying the ability of the body to resist or control infections. Death or illness is a result of these infections, often called opportunistic infections because they turn up when, through impaired immunity, the chance arises.

Origins of the AIDS Virus

Although the precise origin is unknown, and is likely to remain so, it seems probable that a change in nature of a pre-existing virus led to the ability of the HIV virus to invade the human body. Viruses evolve and change, adapting to their environment and establishing themselves in whatever ecological slot is available. The similarity between HIV and other viruses in African monkeys has led to the assumption that the disease originated in that continent. Evidence for the existence of the virus in humans before the early 1970s is unconvincing, but information on the extent of spread through many African countries makes it increasingly clear that it has been present for some time.

Various theories, some of them bizarre and complex, about the transmission of AIDS from Africa to the USA and Europe have been presented. However it seems obvious that such an infectious agent will sooner or later spread to most parts of the globe with the help of modern transport facilities. Those working with any risk group can rapidly identify several possible causes of infection in that group; directly by travel to an area of known infection or indirectly by contact with someone who has. The various modes of transmission considered later, and the possible cross-over of risk groups through people who belong to more than one such group, make spread within a community and between separate communities rapid and easy. More so because of the long incubation period of this disease and the apparent health of infected individuals during this time. There is also the larger group of infected individuals who may not develop the disease despite being infected from a continuous invisible source over a long time. Although in the West the disease emerged first in homosexual men, this merely reflects the lifestyles and activity of that group. There is nothing intrinsic in homosexuality that makes it a unique risk group, as will probably be demonstrated in the next decade. It is probable that AIDS will spread amongst sexually active heterosexuals to a greater extent during this time.

It seems possible that over a period of two decades a similar pattern may emerge in Western countries to that seen in Africa; the impaired transmission during heterosexual intercourse may only mean that it will take longer to emerge.

Groups At Risk

Although the group assumed to have been infected by homosexual intercourse accounts for the largest number of deaths, those who are thought to have obtained the virus by intravenous injection of contaminated material account for 17% of the cases of AIDS in the USA and may well account for more as, previously, homosexual drug users were categorized in the former group. In New York City, 33% of cases of AIDS had occurred in intravenous drug misusers by 1986.

The virus is transmitted by blood to blood contact. This means that it is not spread by aerial droplet method, like the common cold virus, TB or influenza. Similarly, it is not spread by ingestion of contaminated material like salmonella, dysentery, cholera and poliomyelitis. Many widespread epidemic infections due to viruses, bacteria and parasites are spread by bloodsucking insects. There is currently no evidence to show that the AIDS virus has ever been transmitted by this method.

It is, however, transmitted by direct contact with blood or body fluids. This is how it is introduced by anal intercourse, causing absorption through the thin rectal walls and by direct injection into the bloodstream.

Those who have contracted AIDS appear often to have been infected through sexual intercourse, primarily homosexual anal intercourse, but also to a lesser extent heterosexual intercourse. In addition some people have contracted the virus by direct spread through transfusions of infected blood or products of blood. In this latter group are haemophiliacs who have been given contaminated blood products. Although those already infected may well go on to develop the disease, newly infected cases will hopefully be minimal since the introduction of screening for infected donations by the blood transfusion services in most countries. Other body fluids, such as infected semen (as in a case of introduction by artificial insemination in Australia), again exemplify a rare mode of spread. Accidental inoculation of contaminated blood by health workers using needles and other 'sharps' may continue to occur. Reassuringly, very few people experiencing such accidents have contracted enough infection to even register a positive antibody test, far less develop the disease.

Although the great majority of cases of AIDS and deaths from the disease have occurred so far in homosexual men in the United States, this represents only the first, albeit alarming, chapter in the story of the AIDS epidemic. This risk group has taken the brunt of the epidemic so far, simply because its lifestyle is particularly vulnerable to spread of infection. In the USA, and earlier in Africa, there was no warning of the disease and during 1978–1981, when the virus is now known to have been present in both California and New York State, it was spreading rapidly through a sexually active community. Not until 1981 was the disease described and not until much later was the real extent and depth of spread within this group recognized.

Although one would have thought on first consideration that things would now be different, the full extent of spread will take many years to uncover. This is why the enormous death rate projected into the next decade continues to alarm many health professionals. The salutary facts are that, even if behaviour was changed radically in all risk groups today, and no further transmission by any mode happened, then there would still be new cases arising continuously for many years, possibly even decades from now.

Clearly, this sort of change is unlikely for many reasons and spread will continue. The virus is probably here to stay and even with the development of vaccine and drug treatment, cases will continue to develop. The number of cases to be expected is difficult to assess for many reasons. The exact sizes of risk groups, homosexual and drugtaking, are unclear. Without knowing more precisely how many people have been infected by other modes of spread, such as blood transfusion, it is impossible to say how many people will be affected. Most importantly, without understanding the conditions prevailing in sub-Saharan Africa where the disease is endemic in the heterosexual population and appears to be readily spread by sexual activity between men and women, it is impossible to predict whether the same will happen in the industrial countries. Evidence available in Europe and North America is that heterosexual spread is limited. Despite this, slow transmission amongst heterosexuals does occur and over a period of years it is likely to be extensive.

The importance of the spread into the heterosexual risk group is the reduced possibility of control in that community. Whereas homosexuals now recognize themselves as being 'at risk' of catching AIDS, the wider heterosexual community does not.

Heterosexual Spread of AIDS

The identification of AIDS as a 'gay disease' has implications for the heterosexual community. Until the fact that AIDS can potentially be spread by heterosexual activity is understood, young sexually active people will not be aware of the danger and will not take appropriate precautions. The already established infected risk groups in the drug using communities, who are largely heterosexual and sexually active, mix with a group of adults who may have no idea that they are having a sexual relationship with a drug user, far less an infected drug user. In this way, for many reasons and in an invisible manner, the disease will progress into the newer risk group of the heterosexual population. Indeed, the degree of spread already achieved can only be guessed at.

The final risk group of any real importance when considering the intravenous drug using population is those children born to mothers who have acquired the virus by drug use or by sexual contact with an infected person. The possibility that a mother may be infected by a bisexual male is of course important but, as noted above, spread from male to female in this way is limited and therefore case numbers are small at the present time. The majority of infected women becoming pregnant are currently those who have injected drugs themselves. Spread to the child whilst in the uterus appears to occur in approximately half the pregnancies at risk. Progress thereafter is of course dependent on whether or not the baby has been infected. If it has, the outlook appears poor, the child often dying at an early age. Only time will tell about the numbers of survivors and their quality of life. Similarly uncertain is the outlook of the infected mother, as subsequent pregnancies appear to increase the risk of developing the full AIDS disease.

Why Does it Occur in Heroin Users?

As already noted, the prime mode of spread of the AIDS virus in this group is the use of contaminated equipment. In drug using circles, sterile needles and syringes have commonly been in short supply. There are many reasons for this and there is also considerable variation from country to country and from city to city. In some British communities, equipment is available from legal sources such as pharmacists and medical equipment suppliers and, as in many countries, there is no law against possession or purchase of these; they circulate freely. In other areas, prohibition has prevented this supply, often enforced by well-meaning local police drug squads. In addition, until comparatively recently and perhaps still in some areas, the drug user has not been alerted to this particular danger.

For years drug users have been aware of the many and varied dangers of their pastime and amongst these have been infectious diseases such as hepatitis. Also bloodborne transmission of this virus has been noticed frequently in close communities of intravenous drug users but its conse-quences are less severe and most recover, apparently completely. During minor epidemics of hepatitis, people are often more careful about sharing needles and syringes and confine themselves to a restricted circle of appar-ently safe individuals. On a personal level, problems of prevention stem from the fact that the presence of AIDS in this community is comparatively new. In addition, the test which detects the antibody to the virus in the blood of those infected has only been available for a short period, prior to which there was no way of knowing which, if any, of the symptomless drug users were infected.

The final factor making detection and prevention extremely difficult is the long incubation period between acquisition of the virus and onset of symptoms. An infected person may remain symptomless for four or more years, depending on other factors, before developing symptoms of illness. During this period, intravenous drugs may still be used and needles shared widely, thus spreading the infection rapidly. It is easy to see how, in a group of drug users who share equipment, the virus will quickly be transmitted to every individual. Such a group may have many contacts with other smaller or larger groups in the immediate vicinity, or indeed at any distance, and distribution of the virus will be rapid.

In one recent study in Edinburgh, Robertson and Bucknall did a retro-spective testing of samples taken to look for evidence of hepatitis and this showed that the AIDS virus was introduced into a community of drug users in or around August 1983. By March 1985, 50% of over 150 intravenous drug users were known to be infected. In addition, some had no recent blood sample available for testing and if all these were positive, then the total would be 84% positive. This rapidity of spread is likely to occur in any group sharing equipment in a similar way.

The obvious conclusion is that health workers must intervene somehow either to stop needle and syringe sharing or, preferably, to stop individuals injecting heroin at all. Both or either of these measures would immediately reduce to zero the risk of exposure to the AIDS virus by this method. Several UK centres are currently testing the feasibility of providing sterile equipment to drug injectors. Whether the vital health education message will reach the large numbers of drug users rapidly is doubtful. Information should be urgently disseminated, by whatever means deemed appropriate, to educate those drug users at risk although it is not clear which strategies are most likely to deter them from sharing equipment. Even so, the risks posed by such practices to public health are so vast that urgent, if experimental, action should not be delayed.

Prognosis for HIV Positive Individuals

The test currently used to detect whether or not an individual has been infected by the AIDS virus is, for several reasons, inadequate and unsatisfactory. It detects the presence of antibodies to the virus and therefore immediately causes confusion. Logically, the presence of antibodies to the disease indicates that one is immune in the same way as antibodies to measles or rubella viruses imply safety from these diseases. However, the test does not detect the presence or absence of the virus and therefore is only useful in discovering which individuals have been in sufficient contact with the virus to react by producing antibody response. The patient with a positive result to the test for the antibody to the HIV virus can therefore only guess the likely outcome for the future.

Positivity has been examined by testing samples taken from individuals in the past and observing the course of the disease at various times after the first positive result. This method indicated that 10% of those with a positive antibody test would eventually go on to develop AIDS and die. Newer data, however, suggest that this figure may be 30% or greater. However, as positive tests only go back a few years, it is not yet possible to say whether the various surviving groups will develop the disease at a later date or continue to stay fit. In addition, it is of course unknown whether other long term disorders may arise from the presence of the virus in the body. Evidence from the 1986 Paris conference on AIDS has led research workers to be slightly more gloomy about the numbers who may develop the full AIDS syndrome, or even some different manifestation of the disease, and many fear that the majority infected will eventually become ill. Californian researchers have now seen large numbers of people with evidence of brain disorders due to the virus, and the estimates of those developing illnesses of any degree may now be 20–30% rather than the 10% previously anticipated. What will happen to the remaining infected individuals remains one of the great unanswerable questions of the epidemic.

It may be, however, that more sophisticated testing will shortly identify those who have not only antibodies to the virus in their blood but have active live virus replicating in the body. These will be the people, therefore, that one might expect to become ill and to be highly infectious to others, whereas those without live virus may be given a better prognosis. Until these tests are available, one must assume that positivity to the antibody test implies active infection and that the individual might pass on infection by sexual or other means.

A negative result to the test clearly means what it says, but not without some qualification. Rarely, people have developed the disorder in the presence of persistent negative tests and this remains unexplained. In addition, late in the development of the disease, the antibody may be absent from the blood as the individual has lost the capacity to respond to infection by producing antibodies.

Negative tests have the additional caveat that the body may not have had time to develop antibody to a newly acquired infection. Thus, if an individual is tested the day after being exposed to the virus then antibodies are unlikely to be found. Various authorities suggest different times after exposure before one can be sure that the virus has not been acquired. These times vary from three months to one year and indicate the importance of taking precautions against further transmitting the disease until there is absolute certainty, or as near as possible, that the virus has not been acquired.

Ironically, the virus may often be absent from patients dying from AIDS as the cells in which it grows are no longer present. These people therefore are less infectious than a fit and apparently healthy individual who has newly been infected and is still active sexually and socially, as well as being able to use drugs as before. The implications for managing the spread of this disease are clear and the most important of these is that it is impossible to tell by looking at people whether or not they have been in contact with the disease. They may well not know themselves!

Health education is a vital part of managing those unfortunate individuals who have been in contact with the virus. For several reasons, it is important that they understand how their own health can best be preserved, even in the face of a positive result. Firstly, they may not become affected and they are therefore equivalent to those drug users who are negative in that they must immediately avoid further exposure or run the risk of acquiring active infection. Secondly, early results in all risk groups have shown that those who have repeated infection, or other damage to their immune systems such as heroin use, may be more likely to become ill. Those that maintain a correct body weight, eat a good diet and avoid such problems are most likely to remain well. There are good reasons therefore for changing habits, even for those with a positive HIV antibody test. Finally many, if not most, positively tested individuals will hopefully accept their responsibility to others in prevention of spread and make active attempts to avoid exposing and infecting their associates.

Treatment for AIDS

Education is vital. This involves heightened public awareness about AIDS, about sexual activities and dangerous drug using behaviour. At present the only 'cure' for AIDS is prevention. Several highly publicized drugs, such as Suramin, Ribavirin, HPA-23 and lately AZT have not yet been proved effective in treating AIDS. It is probably idealistic to expect that there will be an early solution to this epidemic.

The gay community in the USA, an articulate and powerful force in political and professional life, has been prepared to allow research with drugs and other therapy that has provided the medical establishment with many answers. In addition, they have emphasized the dangers of individuals being stigmatized by the disease and have promoted the sort of sensitivity about confidentiality that has come to be associated with AIDS. This confidentiality is singularly important in a risk group with much to lose in financial, emotional and personal terms if public prejudice is allowed to discriminate against them. Europe had the considerable advantage of being able to learn much from the USA before the disease became established on this side of the Atlantic. There has been an uneasy development of codes of practice and behaviour with reference to confidentiality, treatment, research and atti tudes between the public, the medical establishment and those at risk of contracting the disease. There are obvious examples of gross over-reaction to this, particularly by the mass media and, to a lesser extent, by the public. These have generally been prompted by fear and a lack of understanding of the real threats posed by AIDS. These misconceptions have been com- pounded by the connection between AIDS and minority groups such as homosexuals and drug abusers. Whilst there are and will continue to be rising numbers of individuals suffering the misery and pain of a lethal disease, there may be some reason to feel that through education and public awareness some control over the progress of the disease will emerge in the future to lessen the numbers affected.

Thus, conventional medical care in the widest sense of the term can be applied to a risk group who like to style themselves as unconventional. The application of unconventional care is perhaps a further consideration and alternative measures such as holistic healing, self-help groups, community care and other supports and therapies have been used in America to some effect. Such approaches are worth attempting when all the medical establishment can do is talk about research, vaccines, experimental drugs and what might be available in 1990! The reality is that the great panacea, the vaccine, is of no value to those who are already infected and of little value to those who don't know about AIDS or how it might affect them.

The homosexual community has been able to recognize the enormity of the damage caused by AIDS and to educate themselves appropriately. 'Safer sex' techniques may be useful but will certainly be incomplete in their protection. Whether similar change can be expected in drugtaking behaviour in that emerging risk group remains to be seen. There are several factors which militate against the establishment of the comparable 'safer drugs use' and the type of pressure and educational organization associated with the gay community. Most important perhaps is the illegality of drug use of this sort and the increasingly punitive attitude taken to those involved. Moreover, the position of the drug user in society is one of an outcast and deviant rather than that of an alternative lifestyle. This has given the drug using community a transitory and ethereal quality which defies the researcher, the educationalist and the community. Although there is a continual awareness of the presence of drugs and drug users, it is at the same time covert and often visible only in its consequences. Thus bulging penal establishments, banner headlines in the newspapers and the medical complications all testify to the presence of drug use but in spite of this, there are few self-help groups; there is no 'pro-drug' movement comparable to the well organized gay and lesbian groups in the USA.

Living outside the law and, at least in their drug using behaviour, outside the wider society, drug users are less likely to conform to expectations when it comes to dealing with the AIDS virus. Vaccine may be useless to a group who risk arrest by identifying themselves. Indeed, the great majority of drug users take drugs for many months before encountering an agency or medical person who might advise them about vaccine or other medical measures. Others may never contact such agencies. The availability of hepatitis B vaccine has not prevented what amounts to an epidemic in recent years amongst drug users in many separate centres.

Similarly the application of treatment in conventional forms is notoriously difficult to apply to a risk group under pressure from law enforcement and other establishments. Research, treatment and management of this particular risk group have already proved to be manifestly different from that of more 'conventional' patients.

These difficulties and problem areas are not meant to lead us to the conclusion that drug users cannot, or should not, be treated or that they have any less need or desire to be helped in their plight. But the reality of the situation is that treatment is being withheld, intervention being prevented and close contact being obstructed by society rather than by the drug users themselves. Because society has chosen to disapprove of some drugs and not others, those using the 'bad' drugs are not in a position to represent themselves, to ask for therapy and expect to receive it or to expect the sort of confidentiality reserved for more conventional groups.

This attitude of society to certain types of drug use has led to the expensive drug enforcement operation. The new factor of AIDS poses another serious physical threat to the drug injector and to the community. Increase in 'control' of the drugs problem is unlikely to make things better and may even make the spread of the virus worse. It may even have a counterproductive effect by further alienating drug users from sources of education, information and support thus increasing rather than decreasing ill advised behaviour resulting in spread of infection. Painful as it may be, a lessening of *some* controls is necessary. Drug users need to be drawn into society, not pushed out.

Education remains a critical factor in preventing spread and the ultimate global totals may depend largely on this. Sadly drug education in the past has largely been ineffective and has sometimes been counterproductive. As time goes by, however, the groups which are easy to educate, who pick up information readily either because they are interested or because they are in contact with the correct sources, will be aware of their situation and choose to avoid or alter their potential risk factors. It will become increasingly difficult to make any effect on the pandemic as only those who choose not to listen or to change, or are out of contact for whatever reason, will remain. There will always be the invisible source of infection, the individual who remains undetected either by choice or ignorance.

It does seem that the pattern of the spread of AIDS will change over the years. Whilst the infected members of the major risk groups will continue to become ill and a proportion will undoubtedly continue to die, such groups as blood donation recipients and haemophiliac factor VIII recipients may no longer be at risk to the same extent as previously. Intravenous drug users are already, in some European cities, the worst affected risk group and this carries with it the increased proportion of women infected with the virus. Children born to affected mothers constitute one appreciable risk group and will be an important source of morbidity and death.

AIDS therefore means different problems in different places. In San Francisco it is predominantly confined to male homosexuals with only a small number of intravenous drug users being affected. In New York, however, where over 80% of all cases of AIDS in drug users have been reported, the problem of infected women and consequently infected children is large. Similar patterns are emerging in European centres such as Edinburgh where rising numbers of at risk children are being born reflecting the sizes and activities of the differing risk groups. Although two to three years behind the American experience and therefore represented by positive test results rather than actual cases of disease, Edinburgh demonstrates the New York pattern. Other centres, such as London, exhibit a pattern similar to that seen in California. These variations are not solely dependent on the relative sizes of the risk groups, since there are sizeable gay and drug using communities in many British cities.

In Africa AIDS is a disease of heterosexuals and is attributed to this rather than homosexual behaviour. The place of spread by contaminated needles is unclear. Similarly illicit drug use by injection seems to be unknown. The patterns seen are therefore different and it is clear that the whole sexually active population is at risk in some areas. As many as 10% of those donating blood are found to be positive in Zambia and up to 30% attending sexually transmitted disease clinics. The disease is therefore not one associated only with subgroups or those indulging in illegal or deviant behaviour.

The consequences of all this are perhaps not immediately obvious but to the medical and social work professions at least, it is becoming abundantly clear that both drug misuse and AIDS are multidisciplinary problems of enormous proportions which involve all sectors of society. AIDS is no more a 'gay plague' than any other infectious disease transmitted by blood to blood contact. It will not long be confined to the 'deviant' and conveniently scapegoat risk groups first identified in Europe and America.

7 Prescribing

Prescribing, legislation, control and attitudes have had enormous effects on inappropriate drug use, whether of drugs derived from the legal or illegal market place, and this looks likely to continue or even increase in magnitude. It took several years to recognize that largescale malicious or misguided prescribing contributed to the London drug scene problems of the late 1960s, and that legislation was required to change it. The more subtle and obscure prescribing which continues, not in any way ill motivated but nevertheless damaging, may never be recognized as more than an unavoidable side-effect of managing drug abuse. The fact that this and the subsequent chapter on treatment have been divided may at first seem to be theoretical rather than to represent a different subject. However, prescribing for many reasons plays an important part in maintaining the problem of heroin use in its present situation. This is often but not always related to treatment.

The painfully learned lessons of the early seventies, when the drug dependence clinics prescribed large amounts of opiates, are represented more in the current tight control over prescribing in the North American clinics of today than the comparative freedom of British physicians to prescribe for drug users. This may well lead to problems again as a new group of physicians, namely those doctors specializing in infectious diseases and AIDS, are encountering drug abusers for the first time.

The move from institutional and mainly medical management of drug problems to community care by non-medical personnel and voluntary workers has arisen out of necessity rather than choice. Even so, this shift has assisted in the 'demedicalization' of drug problems and with it, the shift away from emphasis upon punishing policies to the priorities of help for drug-related problems. This move has emphasized that the 'cure' or even the treatment of drug dependence does not lie in the substitution of one drug for another. Newman, with his great experience of drug dependence problems, recognizes this in the statement: 'the challenge for physicians therefore is not achieving abstinence, it is in maintaining it.' Heroin users regularly stop using the drug for variable periods. The crux of the problem is relapse.

Prescribing must be considered because it will probably persist as long as doctors have drugs and as long as patients believe that drugs are what they require. Although there is no doubt that patients often do require drugs and benefit from them, the difficulty is, and always has been, for physicians to decide which patients require which drugs.

This book is not intended to be a reference text. Therefore no attempt will be made to give an encyclopaedic review of types of drugs available via the medical profession. Nevertheless it is useful to consider some historical and ancient examples of drugs and groups of drugs that have been and are being implicated in drug misuse. Apart from heroin, cocaine and cannabis which by statute are not legally available except on rare occasions, the drugs which may be prescribed reflect availability and the prevailing philosophy of the medical profession. It is interesting to note that whilst this latter factor changes from decade to decade, it is also subject to political and geographical constraints. Thus, those commercially prepared drugs available legally or through illegal sources in London will be different from those in New York. Even within one country the drugs in use for legitimate purposes vary from centre to centre and therefore the 'spillage' onto the black market will be different.

Barbiturates

This group of drugs may be described as sedatives or hypnotics and, as such, are members of a much larger group of compounds available for the purpose of tranquillizing or inducing a state of sleep. These are depressant drugs. In a similar way to alcohol, the manifestations of intoxication depend very much on the mental state of the subject and on the circumstances and environment of use. In some people they produce feelings of relief from anxiety or tension, or even euphoria; in others they induce feelings of self pity, anxiety or depression and occasionally some people react with hostility, anger and violent behaviour. Intoxication results in considerable deterioration in complex skills and judgement and is associated with an increased risk of accidents.

The use of barbiturates for medical purposes was at its height in the late 1960s when about 20% of all prescriptions under the National Health Service were for these drugs. The corresponding availability to the illegal market made them possibly the major drug of misuse at that time. Their widespread use and abuse, enshrined in the writings of William Burroughs, were associated with a peak number of deaths in the 1960s which were variously classified as deaths due to suicide, accidental causes, or death due to misadventure, according to local legislation and definitions.

Both tolerance and dependence on barbiturates is achieved fairly rapidly and continued use, like that of many other drugs, is associated with a psychological dependence which often is drug specific. The withdrawal syndrome includes the somatic and psychological features of many drugs of dependence but, more specifically, appears to be associated with often prolonged and dangerous convulsions. The peak of barbiturate misuse was reflected at Lexington Prison in the USA where 18% of those using 'narcotics' in 1955 were severely dependent on barbiturates. In 1961 this had risen to 23% and 35% in 1963.

The voluntary ban (CURB campaign) or limitation on prescribing of barbiturates largely removed, over the following ten years, the misuse of these drugs which some researchers consider to be more damaging than opiates. This was made easier by the development of new effective drugs, such as those in the benzodiazepine group, having similar properties to sedate or as hypnotics but apparently without the major side-effects. The fact that in some centres barbiturates remain available to the drug user is a reflection of the complexity of the interaction between physicians and their patients.

Benzodiazepines

The progression from barbiturates in the 1960s to the discovery at the end of that decade of the benzodiazepine group of drugs allowed for the medical use of a new pharmacological development. Nitrazepam (Mogadon), diazepam (Valium) and chlordiazepoxide (Librium) were rapidly followed by a host of other compounds with similar chemical structures and similar pharmacological properties. The sedative properties of these drugs made them quickly the largest selling drugs in North America and Europe. In 1984, 13 million prescriptions were issued for these drugs in the UK. Their use, however, extended beyond the simple sedative qualities and because they were believed to be safe, they were available to a large part of the community for the relief of anxiety, tension and depression. In a study of 178 Oxford University students in 1983, Golding discovered that 10% of them had recently used drugs of this group. Their anxiolytic (calming) effects had made them popular with the consumer and their apparent low toxicity and safety in overdosage has made them popular with physicians and psychiatrists. The indications for the use of these drugs has extended in recent years to include their use as an anaesthetic agent for minor operative procedures and as a muscle relaxant in various conditions.

Undoubtedly one of the major post-war successes of the pharmaceutical companies, the benzodiazepines represent a significant step forward in the management of many problems and disorders. However, nothing is without its problems and this includes benzodiazepines. A general change in attitudes against medicines as a means of control has highlighted the inappropriate use of these drugs to suppress emotion and anxiety when it arises as a consequence of personal circumstances or difficulties. The sensible recognition that such use of a drug is a temporary solution and may even exacerbate a problem by obstructing the natural course of grief, bereavement or distress has given rise to a rationalization of the use of benzodiazepines. The move to self-help, rather than pharmacological help, can only be regarded as a safer and more appropriate treatment and the widespread application of tranquillizers can be seen in many cases to be controlling a problem rather than treating it.

The second and even more substantial hazard associated with the use of this group of drugs is the identification of a tangible and specific syndrome associated with their continued use. A clear picture has emerged of features of dependence, tolerance and withdrawal, the three classic features of drugs of abuse. Dependence, in common with other drugs, is characterized by a physical and a psychological component and tolerance by the decreased efficacy over a period of prolonged use. In some, this leads to an increased dose being taken and in those who resist this, a return of those symptoms for which the drug was originally taken. Although over short periods of use there seems to be little in the way of detrimental side-effects, at least in some people prolonged use over a period of months is associated with withdrawal symptoms when the drug is discontinued.

Although many of the features of the withdrawal syndrome are similar to other drugs, there appear to be a few drug specific features. Ashton has described the subjective sensations reported to her by her patients as anxiety and apprehension similar to those symptoms which initiate treatment and often attributed to this. However, this can progress to feelings of unreality, distortion in the immediate perception of the environment, 'pins and needles' numbness, unsteadiness in walking or visual disturbance. Paranoid thoughts and feelings of persecution, unreality, agoraphobia and delusions are all included with many more distressing mental and physical complaints. Some features appear to be characteristic of benzodiazepine withdrawal and, although none can be said to be unique to that condition, it is likely that the description of the combined features should identify this condition. Additionally, benzodiazepine withdrawal may continue over many weeks and months especially if the user continues with a reduced dosage. Researchers have tried to answer many of the questions associated with this problem area. Why do most patients have no problems when using these drugs? Why do side-effects go on for so long and often when the blood levels are unrecordable? Is any permanent damage associated with long term use of these drugs or is it reversible? These questions will be answered in time but the recognition of these problems for the time being is the most important development. The use of benzodiazepines over the next decade is likely to show considerable modification, like their predecessors. Long term use is likely to be less desirable and the use of those benzodiazepines with short action, of less value. The shorter the action of the compound the more possible it seems that withdrawal symptoms will develop. Drugs such as lorazepam (Ativan) and triazolam (Halcion) seem therefore particularly problematic. These effects are described in patients given benzodiazepines in pharmacological doses for specific conditions under medical supervision and therefore are related to strengths and dosages within a very confined limit.

Misusers, however, recognize few limits to the use of such drugs and are constrained only by the amount available to them and past experience with the drug. Benzodiazepines, like other drugs, will be taken in doses many times that regarded as normal or even safe. In addition the drug is likely to be taken in combination with other drugs sharing similar properties such as opiates, barbiturates and analgesics.

Knowledge of the effects of 5–10 mg of Valium taken over a period may be of less immediate importance when faced with those using 100–150 mg per day in association with other drugs. Clearly the benzodiazepine withdrawal story will be an important factor for those dealing with people complaining of withdrawal symptoms from a variety of legal and illegal drugs. A knowledge of all the drugs being used up to the time of cessation of use is vital.

Amphetamines

These are stimulant drugs often known colloquially as 'pep-pills' or 'speed'. Originally made synthetically in 1887, these drugs were first used medically during the 1930s when their psychoactive activity was first recognized. During the Second World War they were distributed to military personnel and industrial workers in many countries as an aid to overcome drowsiness while doing dull or repetitive tasks. They were issued to commandos and airmen on long distance missions and included in first aid and survival kits. After the war, stocks were released to civilians which had an important effect on the development of amphetamine misuse in many countries. Progressive changes in medical attitudes led to a voluntary restriction of the use of these drugs. This had a big impact on black market supplies. In spite of this amphetamines, often in the form of amphetamine sulphate powder, are still widely available from illegal sources.

Physical dependence on amphetamines is considered to be less than other drugs of abuse although rapid development of tolerance, with increased dosage, is common. The drug may be taken orally or intravenously in doses of 20–160 mg many times a day and has a rapid intense effect of short duration. Episodes of intensive use are common over days or weeks, followed by a 'crash' in which there is prolonged sleep, depression and apathy. The experience of amphetamine psychosis may be associated with paranoid delusions, compulsive repetitive behaviour, jaw grinding and other distressing symptoms.

The popularity of amphetamines has come and gone over the decades of the twentieth century. From the enormous post-war problems up to the end of the fifties, various countries recognized an amphetamine abuse problem. In 1954 in Japan, there were between 500,000 and 600,000 users of these drugs, 300,000 of whom administered it intravenously. Legislation in the USA in 1966 stopped the enormous legal trade in these drugs and the millions of amphetamine tablets which were available without prescription.

The ability to synthesize this drug locally has always allowed those involved with the illicit supply to manufacture it close to the point of sale and therefore avoid the dangers and risks associated with the importation of natural compounds such as heroin, cocaine or cannabis. The use of amphetamines by heroin users is a longstanding combination taken intravenously in the same way as cocaine and heroin are often taken together, providing a short intense euphoria followed by a longer lasting opiate effect. The use of cocaine is increasingly popular in North America whereas the problems of availability in Europe have encouraged more amphetamine use. In many areas the rather misguided prescription of injectable amphetamines and similar drugs has established a requirement in the drug using community for this type of substance and it seems that only now in the 1980s are Methedrine, Ritalin, Preludin, Filon and others becoming restricted medically and, in some cases, by companies ceasing their commercial manufacture.

Many groups and sub-cultures have had a place for the use of these drugs, from the obese and bored to the wild and the dangerous. The youthful abuse of the 1960s in London, Stockholm and New York has given way to a more steady, less fluctuating availability based less on legitimate prescriptions and more on illegal manufacture. Regional variations continue to exist; Stockholm still has an amphetamine problem greater than that of heroin, the intravenous users of which have now been found to include some with HIV (AIDS) virus infection. In the UK however, intravenous amphetamine use is secondary to that of heroin and in New York pushed further down the list of drugs taken intravenously by the enormous preference for cocaine. Stimson reported in his 1982 book that in 1969, 44% of London drug users interviewed had or did use amphetamines whilst a 1986 report from Bucknall confirms continuing use in 41% of those interviewed in his Scottish research.

Interestingly, in the later report, barbiturate use had dropped from 83% to 22% but the other groups remained similar with the exception of newer drugs such as buprenorphine which was not available in 1969.

Buprenorphine (Temgesic)

As technology continues to progress in every field of human interest, the pharmaceutical industry year by year develops and refines its armoury of compounds. Old or obsolete drugs are abandoned and those with more useful and hopefully less toxic effects are introduced in their place. Attitudes and public acceptability have much to do with what is useful and acceptable, especially when side-effects are present and when behaviour altering or psychoactive properties exist.

Buprenorphine, an opiate type pain killer, was introduced in the 1970s in the UK and became available on general prescription in an oral form in the early 1980s. It is taken by being dissolved under the tongue and has a much longer duration of action than morphine. It is thought to have a low dependence potential. Unlike most narcotic pain killing drugs its effects are not reversed by naloxone, the specific antidote used in overdosage of opiates. Because of its opiate and opiate antagonist properties, it may precipitate mild opiate withdrawal in those addicted or using high doses of opiates. As it is active only when taken under the tongue or by injection, overdosage is rare and reported to be less dangerous than other opiates. However, in the few years of its availability in the UK, it has become established as a drug of potential abuse for those choosing to take it inappropriately.

The drug user may take it orally to reduce the requirement for illegal opiates or inject the tablets or solution intravenously with a resulting narcotic type of experience. Its interaction with other opiates is observed by those using both and its ability to reduce the effect of heroin is understood by drug takers. Nevertheless, in common with other opiates from legal sources, it is much sought after especially when illegal supplies are restricted. Its theoretical value as an agent to reduce requirement for opiates and to stabilize dependence problems has led, at times, to ill advised prescribing under conditions difficult to control, as described by Robertson (1986).

Dihydrocodeine, Codeine, Dextropropoxyphene

These preparations are chemically related to morphine but with a variable potency usually less profound than the parent compound. Methadone is a similar synthetic opiate and many other examples are available in European and North American countries. The examples discussed here are used not because they are the most powerful or those with the most marked effects, but because they represent drugs freely available on prescription and therefore in common use. In addition, because of this comparatively free availability, they represent a group of pharmaceutically prepared drugs accessible to the contemporary drug user. The part they have to play in mortality and damage to health is at present understated.

All these preparations are used in a useful and appropriate way for their pain relieving effects. As with other opiates, they have a depressant effect on the central nervous system and although this is no danger if used independently and in controlled doses, taken in excessive quantities or in combination with other such drugs they are potentially lethal. As Ghodse (1985) has indicated, the role of these and other drugs in combination may account for many episodes of death in heroin users and the sporadic nature of deaths attributed to this cause may, in some cases, be accounted for by a sudden supply of such drugs being mixed with illegal heroin. The inexperienced heroin user may think little of the dangers of taking a 'shot' of heroin in combination with or following on the ingestion of some harmless looking pain killers whose effect seems to be minimal.

The ill-advised or uncontrolled prescribing of drugs of all types has, therefore, a marked effect on the illicit market and although there has been a change since the sixties when the 'drug scene' in the UK and Europe was largely dependent on legal sources of heroin, amphetamines and other drugs, the present large supplies of illicit heroin should not obscure the enormous abuse of 'legal' drugs which continues to this day. The rather obvious effects and side-effects of barbiturates, Ritalin, Methedrine and Dexedrine may be less apparent but the harmful and lethal effects of the newer drugs of abuse may be more obvious if we looked for them. As new compounds are discovered and promoted and new claims are made for their beneficial effects, their inevitable abuse will follow. Prescribed drugs always provide a backdrop to the drug scene. They are always available as an alternative when other sources are temporarily suspended and for that reason, careful consideration of their potential for misuse should precede their supply.

Substitution Therapy

For almost 20 years those involved with provision of services for problem drug users have grappled with the problems of prescribing alternative drugs with a view to effecting a 'cure'. For many reasons, there has been an ebb and flow of opinions, and various claims made for different types of drugs as agents which might either cure or make recovery less difficult. Until comparatively recently, the few days after cessation of drug use dominated most people's thoughts and therapy was often directed to alleviating these early withdrawal symptoms. The assumption was that once over the painful and miserable few days of discomfort, a new resolve would carry the patient on from there to maintain abstinence. Unfortunately, clear and recurrent observations by all involved with this rather simplistic approach make it obvious that the majority of such individuals (like many problem drinkers) frequently return for a further course of such treatment, indicating a failure to achieve its objective.

Repeated failures of this nature, either in one individual or a group of patients, often lead the therapist to despair and consequent withdrawal of involvement. This may lead to deteriorating relationships with such patients and subsequent reinforcement of the failure in the eyes of the therapist.

These problems, very familiar in most medical practices, may be seen as a lack of understanding of both therapist and patient. To imagine that the only reason why an individual will not stop using a damaging drug like heroin is because of the few days of discomfort is to misunderstand the basic nature of drug use. Individuals use drugs for a wide variety of reasons. These include social, domestic and employment issues as well as personality, environment and as a result of previous experiences with drugs of one sort or another. Many researchers have described problems leading to drugs misuse but the majority would now agree that there is no one factor which causes illicit drug use and therefore there is unlikely to be one treatment or therapy which will effect a cure (Fazey 1977, Plant 1981).

The establishment of a drug-free state or the process of detoxification therefore must not be confused with a cure or even successful treatment. Cure is something which can only be retrospective in that relapse into drug use may occur at any time. After a period of some years abstinence, an individual may look back and speculate about the cause of his change of behaviour. He may even be prepared to isolate a point in time and an event, or series of events, which brought about abstinence. Most however, with the memory of many attempts and failures before final cessation of drugs use, will be unwilling to isolate a single point in time or a single event as the cure or the time when they experienced recovery.

Spontaneous Abstinence Complicating Treatment

Further complicating the underlying philosophy of treating drug misuse is the awareness in both therapist and patient of spontaneous abstinence without any recognized therapy. Most people who have used drugs, and even drugs which are considered to be highly dependence-producing, will describe long periods of use interspersed with short or longer periods of reduced intake of the drug. In addition most individuals will have had episodes of days or weeks when no drug has been taken at all. Such abstinent periods may be attributed to non-availability of the drug or to non-requirement for the drug and the latter may be due to any number of social or environmental factors. The presence or absence of family or social problems may preclude drug use or divert the attention of the drug user from his usual behaviour. The acquisition or loss of a loved one may modify behaviour, as may the requirement for solving a personal or domestic problem. Clearly any such life event may effect permanent abstinence or conversely, if the experience is an unpleasant one, the relapse to the drug using state. It is important however to see the behaviour of drug use as variable from day to day and from week to week as it is from person to person. A drug user may therefore describe in retrospect many periods of prolonged abstinence related or unrelated to therapy. He may equally well describe periods of prolonged or exceptionally heavy drug use and relate these episodes to life events of a detrimental or unpleasant nature.

Similarly, different individuals will describe patterns of drug use and each person will give a profile of drug use which is personal and unique.

Applying Therapy to Individual Profiles

As in other areas of therapeutics, and especially in treatments for behavioural or personality disorders, the requirement is for a therapy suitable to the individual at the time when help is sought. People, being what they are, will require a variety of approaches and one individual will even require a variety of types of intervention at different stages in life. It is therefore unlikely that one type of therapy or intervention will be effective for everyone, even though the problems seem identical. It is unlikely also that the same therapy repeated at different times will be effective even in the same individual.

There is a need therefore for a range of agencies and provisions and for a careful selection of the type of intervention most appropriate for that problem or individual personality.

Methadone Maintenance

The traditional and acceptable solution for many has been the provision of an alternative opiate to remove the requirement to take illegal drugs. This has the obvious advantage of releasing the drug user from the criminal world of illicit black markets, stealing to provide cash to buy drugs and the violence and aggression surrounding the drug scene. It has also the potential advantage of allowing the individual the opportunity to leave the environment or at best the company of other drug users. The attractiveness of a maintenance supply of an alternative drug such as methadone is further clear if one believes that, in a controlled state, the drug user will make use of facilities provided to understand his problems and to look for and strive to achieve lasting solutions. Finally, and to many people crucially important, the establishment of a controlled state and one over which society has influence reduces the damage caused to people and property previously at risk. A comparatively new and compelling argument to reinforce this is the damage being done to drug users and their contacts by the spread of AIDS. The economic cost to the community of treatment for victims will far outweigh the cost of maintaining the entire population of heroin users on a drug like methadone.

Before examining the problems associated with methadone maintenance as a line of intervention, it is important to consider further the rationale behind its use and the expectations of therapists when they recommend it.

Having established that detoxification is a peripheral issue in long term treatment, and a maintenance programme by definition will not run into this problem, we can move on to consider whether or not cure is part of this type of treatment at all and, if not, what measure of success is sought. Obviously establishing a steady state in which the patient is receptive is one achievement. Removing the damaging effects of adulterated illicit heroin is another. Protecting society is an important third attainment. This, therefore, might be enough to justify this approach.

Problems with Maintenance Prescribing

The beneficial effects outlined above are attractive and often this type of sanctuary is welcomed by the disordered drug user who may be in a distressed state. The provision of a long term drug of dependence cannot, however, be seen as a cure for drug problems. To provide an alternative legal supply may be seen for what it is by therapists and health workers, namely avoiding the issue rather than treating the disorder. The progressive disillusionment with maintenance therapy however is not so much a recognition of an illogical approach as an appreciation of the practical difficulties of administering and delivering the system to a group of individuals looking for something more appropriate. That drug users on maintenance therapy have continued to use illicit drugs is now clear. Over half the drug users attending the New York drug treatment programmes have been exposed to the AIDS virus. Some of these acquired the infection before involvement in the therapy but others continued to inject street heroin as well as using the legal supply of methadone. Resale of methadone is known to occur and the money received for this may well be used to buy illegal drugs. The therapist may therefore be providing funds for the purchase of black market supplies.

Maintenance of a stable state undoubtedly has its advantages but it is unclear whether a stable state induced by continuous drugs use allows one to contemplate and resolve the very complex psychological issues of dependence. The continued provision of an opiate drug in the maintenance programme provides a stability to which most drug users must be unaccustomed, relying usually on an irregular and unpredictable black market. So continuous drug administration is likely, for the reasons outlined above, to result in the long term use of more drugs than in the untreated state. The average daily amount of opiate taken will quickly overtake that used when dependent on illegal sources in all but the very heavy user.

Withdrawing from use of the alternative drug is notoriously difficult for all these reasons and therefore leads to prolongation of therapy. One practical difficulty is the fact that methadone remains in the body for a comparatively long time. This causes protracted withdrawal symptoms of a more severe nature than those associated with heroin. Prolonged therapy has given rise to the large numbers of opiate dependent patients still after many years attending clinics for daily provision of methadone. Many of these drug users may have stopped using drugs years before if they had not received such prescriptions. Evidence suggests that many drug users 'mature out' of drug use and that cessation of involvement with illegal drugs may well be a natural development which is impaired by a maintenance programme. Similarly, many young people reduce their alcohol consumption during their twenties and thirties (Plant, Peck and Samuel 1985). Social and medical control, such as maintenance prescribing, applied to these individuals would be as unacceptable as it would be impossible to administer due to sheer numbers. This latter reason has been one of the deciding factors in the movement of the medical establishment away from maintenance therapy. The philosophical issues, however, remain unresolved and because of this, represent a threat that this therapy, which is not really a therapy at all, will re-emerge as a solution to the problem of AIDS in intravenous drug users.

Non-maintenance Methadone Prescription

As a logical progression from continuous provision but still with the assumption that treatment is being used to overcome side-effects of heroin withdrawal, methadone in reducing doses is currently advocated by many doctors and therapists. The current UK recommendation for management of heroin users issued to doctors by the Department of Health and the Scottish Home and Health Department relies heavily on the prescription of methadone to achieve abstinence. Whilst it is accepted that short courses should be attempted and the drug-free state achieved quickly, prescribing another drug as the best line of management reflects the persistent attitude of the medical profession to drugs and treatment of drug misuse.

The belief that management of the withdrawal syndrome is making a major contribution is a further inadequacy.

Conclusion

Much is unclear about the value or dangers of prescribed drugs. This chapter however has attempted to demonstrate the presence of these substances and their availability to those using illegal drugs such as heroin.

It must be clear that the provision of legal drugs may often be damaging and may at times provide an income when resold on the 'black market'. Table 7.1 shows the street value of prescribed drugs in Edinburgh in 1986 and how a prescription for one hundred of any of these may be worth much to the recipient.

The dangers of prescribed drugs in overdosage or in combination with illegal drugs are enormous and may account for many deaths attributed solely to heroin.

Table 7.1

Drug	Street price
Methadone linctus 30 mls (30 mg)	£10.00
Diconal (dipipanone) 1 tablet	£6.00
Temgesic (buprenorphine) 1 tablet	£3.00
DF118 (dihydrocodeine) 1 tablet	30p
Valium (diazepam) 10 mg 1 tablet	20p
Valium (diazepam) 5 mg 1 tablet	10p
Halcion (triazolam) 1 tablet	10p

Medical practitioners are trained in the use of pharmaceutical preparations and although they are aware of side-effects and toxic levels, the deliberate concealing of amounts taken and other drugs used make this difficult to supervise. More important however is the dominant position of the prescription in the management of heroin users. Both doctor and patient may believe sincerely that the provision of a drug or drugs is the main part of therapy and therefore any consultation is principally about the type, dose, strength and length of course of medicine to be taken.

It may be that this process inhibits treatment of the real disorder, which has little to do with drugs.

8 Treatment

Since the use and misuse of opiates became more than a small problem isolated mainly amongst those with access to pharmaceutical supplies of heroin or morphine, publications and information sources on the subject have been surprisingly evasive about treatment. Claims for successful therapies have in recent years been less forthcoming and the widely idealized 'British system' which centred round the supply of an alternative drug, thus preventing the establishment of a reliance on illegal sources, has fallen into disuse. An increasing number of books on the subject of drug problems have concentrated on the examination of the drugs used, their pharmacology and effects and the behaviour and damage consequent on their use. Many describe the history of previous decades of drug misuse and the events of the late seventies and early eighties which have led to the present situation. The majority are strangely silent on the subject of treatment, which is usually included in a chapter of lists of helping agencies and brief descriptions of the type of help on offer.

Just why so little attention is paid to treatment of substance abuse and why so few agencies, including the main focus of therapy in medical centres, have produced information may at first be unclear. Problems have undoubtedly arisen in assessing what is being done, what effect it has and whether the effect can be shown to be the cause of change, if there has indeed been any change in the individual's behaviour. The majority of people who have misused a drug such as heroin and have come to the attention of an agency, have been in contact with a number of agencies. Claims for success have to take into account previous treatments received by an individual, which may well have had a delayed effect. Trying to decide when, after the onset of abstinence, cure has been achieved has bedevilled workers in substance abuse therapy for many years. Even the longest established and best organized therapeutic programme experiences unpredictable results and therefore lacks prognostic indicators which might show which patient can be expected to do better as a result of a specific type of intervention.

Long term follow-up studies of groups of drug users have shown that there is some correlation between prolonged abstinence from drug use and length of stay in certain types of therapeutic programmes or length of time attending certain clinics. Unfortunately, no information is available to confirm or deny the possibility that these individuals were selected by whatever process brought them into the therapy and were therefore a group who would be expected to do well in the long term without any treatment. The individuals defaulting or not enrolling in therapy may be the ones who would be unlikely to benefit anyway by virtue of their personality, or their special problem.

There may therefore be subgroups within the whole population of heroin users who might, over a period of time, pursue a better or a more destructive path. Examples of this are clearly seen in a number of areas of drug misuse where different groups perform differently in relation to a certain problem. Those who persistently inject drugs might be expected to develop different problems from those who rarely or never inject. Those who share needles and syringes will expose themselves to the risk of hepatitis or AIDS whereas those not sharing will not risk acquiring these viruses by that route. Those with social or family support may be expected to do better than those without. The problem with assessing therapy therefore has been to pin down what it is that therapy is trying to achieve and in what type of individual.

Logically one might state that the object of therapy is to achieve abstinence. If, however, abstinence is transitory, has the therapy been unsuccessful? If the abstinent period is one month, or six months or even one year, would one consider the treatment to be effective or satisfactory or would such a relapse at any time in the future denote failure? If, in a similar way, the individual continues to abuse drugs in the same way as before therapy but at a future date abstains, is it reasonable to assume that the therapy might have had some influence on that outcome? The therapy might not affect drug intake at all but in some way alter behaviour to make it less destructive or to make the outcome less damaging to society or the user's immediate environment. Therapy in that case might be considered to have improved the situation or an aspect of the situation and therefore be beneficial to patient, family and community.

The possibility that, in many individuals, heroin or any drug problem is a transitory phase further complicates the evaluation of long term outcome studies of groups of misusers. Many workers observe such episodes in the lives of individual adolescents and clearly many young people abuse drugs who never came to the attention of medical or agency workers of any kind. Just how to recognize these individuals in a study group of drug users has, so far, eluded researchers, but the knowledge that many heroin users give up with no medical or other professional help compromises satisfactory planning of outcome studies.

Unfortunately, this sort of information can be detrimental in different ways. It can lead professionals to the conclusion that because one drug user can abstain and remain drug free with no obvious help, everyone can. It also can lead drug users or professionals to conclude that because one individual can use a drug like heroin and avoid any serious consequences then others will do so. Neither of these conclusions is accurate and both obstruct understanding and therefore investigation of a complex situation. In addition this sort of logic has been used by the medical establishment to rationalize the withdrawal of attempts to engage drug users in treatment.

There are many reasons why these questions have not been answered in the years since heroin misuse became common. In many cases it is clear that they cannot be answered. However, it is vital that they be considered before logical intervention can be planned. If one is expecting, eventually, to effect abstinence in all cases, then it will very quickly be possible to assess the effectiveness of the treatment. If, however, one accepts that complete abstinence in all cases is unlikely or too much to expect, then the level of success must be defined in order that the therapy can be assessed or evaluated. Increasingly institutions and agencies are taking a pragmatic approach to therapy and accepting that the relapse rate will be high. Improvement in other areas might be expected, changes in behaviour, modifications in drug use, improvements in socialization or reduction in criminality. All these might be considered to be a beneficial outcome of therapy and therefore a success, albeit partial.

In this chapter traditional therapy will be considered, followed in the next by a discussion of new ideas or directions in treatment and how these changes might be expected to come about. Throughout it must be remembered that reference to heroin misusers, or drugtakers, includes a wide variety of individual types and drug-related problems. A 16 year old heroin user taking a few milligrams of heroin per day, or even per week, represents quite a distinct challenge from a 35 year old veteran of long term multidrug misuse who has experiences, good and bad, of many more doctors and workers than the present therapist. This must be borne in mind when considering why therapy may or may not work. The 16 year old may have a simple solution to his or her problem which has nothing to do with clinical psychologists, psychiatrists or social workers, as indeed, on a rare occasion, may the 35 year old. The important prerequisite for the discussion therefore is the recognition that everyone is involved with treatment and on occasions everyone can be successful. Family, neighbours, friends, professionals and society have an important role to play.

Traditional or Conventional Aims

Primary Prevention

Central to recent Government policy on drug misuse has been the concept of primary prevention, that is prevention of the initial onset of drugtaking. This is the ideal solution and would presumably be the most cost-effective policy to pursue. Most people have a role to play in primary preventive measures. Agencies such as the Scottish Health Education Group and the now reformed Health Education Council can develop strategies and direct funds to educate and bring important information to the notice of those at risk. However, the concept of this type of education presupposes that we know or understand the causes of drug problems. Without the knowledge of what we are trying to prevent or what causes it, education and information dissemination is, at best, a shot in the dark. Furthermore, such intervention might just as logically have detrimental consequences. Outlining previously unknown possibilities may induce experimentation and information which is incorrect or misleading may discredit the information source in the eyes of the recipient. Education clearly always has a role to play and is a major requirement of any sophisticated or civilized society. It does, however, have to be the correct information and it does have to be presented and received by the correct individuals. The ideal requirement is to understand the causal factors and those circumstances which are likely to make things better or worse.

There are many reasons why a national campaign aimed at primary preventive measures may be an attractive and cheap approach to combating drug misuse. Sadly such exercises are unlikely to have much impact on such a complex problem. Local educational campaigns may be an additional mode of disseminating information and already are active in promoting simple messages relevant to local needs and problems. Agencies working close to problems may have more success and easier access to drug users. Experience in Europe and America has recently shown the requirement for specific local information and education. This is principally because drug misuse and its consequences have many manifestations and may be quite different in even closely situated centres.

Since the late 1960s the focus of attention of treatment for drug misuse, and in particular opiate misuse, has been the psychiatric sector of the National Health Service in the United Kingdom, and designated drug treatment centres usually administered by psychiatrists in North America and Europe. In addition there has been an involvement of independent (or private) practitioners who, whilst subscribing generally to the medical model of treatment have, for reasons examined later, changed less with the times than their colleagues.

Initial confidence that at least in the UK, the designated drug treatment clinics would cope adequately and in a uniform way with the problems as they arose in different areas, has given rise to a fragmented and inconsistent service. Varying attitudes and philosophies throughout the country have resulted in widely different provisions of services varying from inclusion of drug misusers in general psychiatric clinics where doctors and nurses have no special training or laboratory facilities at their disposal, to long established dinosaurs of substance abuse, the methadone maintenance programmes seen more commonly in the USA than in Europe. The establishment of cohorts of drug users in such programmes has led over the years to an anomalous situation of research emanating from centres providing this sort of facility. The study of groups of long term maintenance patients, most of whom may have been dependent on drugs for many more years than those who never entered this type of therapy, may provide information of value only in the understanding of this group and in no way representative of the present day new recruit to heroin.

Methadone

This synthetic opiate, which is presented in a preparation which can only be tolerated orally, has been the centre of much interest in heroin addiction therapy for many years. Its use can be divided into these categories:

Short term – detoxification
Long term – maintenance
High dose – (narcotic blockade) maintenance.

Short Term Methadone

Although considered as a group, these three types of therapy embody quite different philosophies to treatment. The first represents a quick substitution during the period of maximum crisis in the life of an opiate user; to immediately remove the requirement to obtain illegal drugs and to rapidly achieve a stable and controlled situation. This is followed by a rapid reduction, over a period of days or at the most weeks, of the substituted drug to achieve a drug-free state at the end of this time. Having achieved this, appropriate support should follow the patient through to a more stable existence not involving drug taking.

The superficial attractions of such a regime are easy to see and this formed the basis of the National Guidelines on the Management of Drug Abusers issued in the UK in 1984. Although this may well work in a minority of cases, it requires close attention to the other factors which are to be brought into play to prevent relapse. Such a short course implies that the only thing preventing long term abstinence from heroin is the difficulty presented during the withdrawal phase. It takes no account of the many and various factors causing continuation of opiate misuse, the least of which is withdrawal symptomatology. In a unit with an established support system for intervening with the life and socialization of drug users, this short term substitution treatment has a limited application as an adjunct to treatment, but in an uncontrolled, non-specialist situation it often becomes a major problem for patient and therapist. The carefully selected patient who, for personal reasons, is well motivated and determined to achieve abstinence, will often proceed satisfactorily to the drug-free state in a matter of a few weeks, or even less, and results can be satisfying for both patient and family. In the event of further illegal drug use, the same intervention may be effective in future.

Experience shows however that this happy scenario is not representative of most cases. Relapse is common, if not the normal situation, and repeated courses of a reduction regime are similarly effective at the time, but of short term benefit. In addition, manifest manipulation of such prescribing is enough to alarm the most enthusiastic doctor or therapist. Repeated requests for substitute drugs to overcome real or perceived withdrawal symptoms can quickly lead to a situation where prescriptions are almost continuous and often illegal drugs, or those from another legitimate source, fill the gap between prescriptions. Rules and guidelines, based often on the tolerance of the practitioner, are laid down to establish how far he is prepared to negotiate prescribing therapies and attempts are made to keep within these boundaries.

Problems, therefore, are considerable in the practical management of alternative prescribing and perhaps consideration of the logic behind this intervention is best explained here. To overcome and stabilize behavioural problems is attractive and these are usually directly related to the effects of a psychoactive drug or to the peripheral need for illegal activities to subsidize the costs of providing an expensive drug. Unless the continued provision of an alternative drug is to be contemplated, then the prescription must stop sooner or later and, for many reasons, this should be sooner.

For one reason or another, treatment of heroin abuse in the minds of many drug users and many doctors begins, and ends, with the prescription of an alternative drug such as methadone. This is probably because of the traditional obsession of both groups with the withdrawal phase of recovery rather than the underlying causes of drugtaking. The withdrawal syndrome is a cluster of psychological and physical symptoms perceived by an individual during the time when administration of a drug stops. That they are largely psychological is often accepted by drug user as well as therapist. Physical symptoms may include up to 50 separate sensations or bodily disorders. The most common and distressing however are sleeplessness, anxiety, apprehension, abdominal discomfort, running nose, diarrhoea and sweating. If drug intake has been excessive or prolonged then these are likely to be severe and if intake is minimal they may be absent completely. Many heroin users take the drug intermittently or so seldom as to experience no withdrawal between doses. Fatal consequences from withdrawal from opiates are virtually unknown. Withdrawal symptoms, therefore, can sensibly be managed by gradual reduction of the illegal substances followed by provision for the minimal symptoms experienced thereafter. This, however, does not always comply with the expectations of the drug user or his family and therefore it is fundamental to the argument.

Long Term Methadone

Recognizing that many drug users are unable to refrain from drug use following withdrawal, the introduction of methadone provides a comparatively safe alternative drug. That such chronic drug dependent individuals were unlikely to ever become drug-free was something that seemed logical to those in the late 1960s and early 1970s who were involved with increasing numbers of heroin users. In 1966, Paulus in Canada described the use of 'prolonged methadone withdrawal' during which time a narcotic user might be 'maintained on methadone until such time as he, or she, can either function without a narcotic, or other factors warrant discontinuation of medication . . .'. This early evaluation of methadone in low dosage (up to 40 mg daily) was followed over the ensuing decade by many appraisals of its values. The Nixon administration of the early seventies was much impressed by the results of an ambitious plan to put massive funds into the provision of such projects. The results of 'methadone for everyone' showed a dramatic reduction in the success rate. Similar disillusionment with methadone has followed and the recognition of its dangers and potential problems has changed its application from a treatment in itself to being recognized as a control over an impossible situation or, at best, an adjunct to psychological and social restructuring. Current American initiatives by the Reagan administration are again providing funding for methadone programmes. In the light of the existing AIDS problems, control is seen to be mandatory although treatment remains controversial.

High Dose Narcotic Blockade

The work of Dole and Nyswander was influential in the early methadone enthusiasm. Considering heroin dependence to be a metabolic disease and that 'addict traits' are a consequence not a cause of drug use, this therapy required large doses of methadone (often over 100 mg per day) to block the effects of heroin and therefore to obviate the value of taking additional illegal drugs.

The early success of this therapy was not duplicated when applied to an unselected group and its results may partially represent the selection of drug users who had no psychiatric illness, used no other drugs and had used heroin for at least four years. This group has subsequently been shown to be most likely to stop using heroin even with little or no treatment.

Whatever the reasons, the failure to accept the theory that there was a metabolic basis for addiction and the difficulty in applying and controlling such a regime has meant that high dose therapy is no longer in general use.

Much resistance to methadone programmes has been stated since their original inception. Many authorities on methadone maintenance remain quite committed to their views. Bratter (1984) reaffirms his statement of 1974:

'Scientifically until many of the medical issues regarding the short and long term physiological effects are answered, methadone maintenance remains an unproven enigma. Medically, to subject approximately 100,000 human beings to a potent chemical without proper controls is malpractice of the most insidious sort. Legally, to imprison marijuana smokers and heroin addicts as criminally dangerous while concurrently maintaining that methadone addicts are law abiding, is a travesty of justice. Philosophically, to confuse deliberately the concepts of 'treatment' with 'social control' is fraudulent. Psychologically, to convince addicts that there is a mystical metabolic disorder and that they must remain dependent on a potential poison rather than to strive for their autonomy, is a conspiracy. Ethically, any conspiracy which places people in 'no win' situations and militates against their growth and development must be considered a criminal act!'.

Naltrexone (Trexan)

This drug, available for some time in the USA, has provided an alternative treatment for opiate dependence. It is an antagonist which blocks the effects of opiates on the body. It does not, however, abolish the craving for narcotics. Taken together with other opiates it competes with these drugs and can cause acute withdrawal symptoms, as soon as five minutes after administration. It must therefore be taken after detoxification.

The competition between drugs can be reversed by sufficiently large doses of narcotics and therefore patients taking naltrexone should be warned about the possibility of overdosage if they attempt to override the blockade.

Early studies were disappointing, many patients opting out of treatment before any conclusion could be reached. Subsequent studies have shown better results when ancillary services such as behavioural and family therapy were also available (Kosten & Kleber 1984). It seems to be most useful in discouraging impulsive narcotic use, an important cause of relapse.

Far from being the panacea for the treatment of opiate users, naltrexone has additional side-effects. It must be used with caution by patients with liver damage or recent hepatitis and careful monitoring is required. Its place in the treatment of heroin use is therefore not established, although great interest is likely to be shown in its use to prevent relapse in controlled users or those achieving long abstinent periods.

Preparation for Abstinence

Success or failure balances very much on expectation of the likely benefits of therapy or the ease with which results are achieved. The fact that the withdrawal phase is seen as a hurdle to be overcome, is a direct precursor to failure. The belief that this is the only problem is naive and the assumption that all will be well after symptoms have subsided is obstructive to progress. Most drug users will have experienced the disappointment of finding that, having achieved abstinence, nothing has changed. The desires and temptations to use the drug are still there and no new ability to cope with this has been developed.

If the withdrawal phase is indeed a red herring, then it explains why failure rates are high in a treatment regime aiming only at achieving abstinence. The provision of a detoxification facility at whatever type of institution or centre is therefore unlikely to show impressive results. This is indeed the experience of many hospitals and short term centres, where maximum effort and consequently maximum attention is placed on the physical and psychological problems of those first few hours and days following the last administration of the drug. In the view of the therapist and patient, failure at this stage represents total failure and often causes confusion and disappointment. The lessons of twenty years or more of such experiences are slow to penetrate the providers of funds or services for drug users. The assumptions remain that it is not a condition amenable to treatment or that it is not a medical condition at all and therefore does not merit resources or medical attention.

Similar conclusions may be that drug users themselves are resistant to treatment and that they, for reasons not understood, do not wish to be cured or helped. How often is it said, with some degree of relief, that there is nothing anyone can do if the drug user does not want to help himself? The assumption underlying all these statements and ideas is that the treatment would be excellent but the patient is unsuitable or unwilling to cooperate. How many surgeons would get away with a failure rate greatly exceeding success rate by providing the logic that the operation is successful but the patients always seem to die?

Later on in this chapter it is noted that some of this illogical process is being eroded and that for the first time therapies are changing to suit the requirement of the patient. It is important to recognize that preparation for any type of therapy, even simple detoxification, must be fundamental to successful treatment. The individual entering a simple regime must understand what it is likely to achieve and what it is not likely to achieve. If it is understood that the same pressures and environmental strains will apply after therapy, then disappointment might not be so great. If the patient acknowledges that failure will not be the fault primarily of the therapy and that the patient has at least as much influence as the therapist on success, then chances must be improved. If it is recognized that success is not necessarily instantaneous and that experiences can be built upon, then the further use of drugs after the therapeutic experience may not necessarily cause the patient to abandon all that has been learned and to assume that all is again lost.

In short, therefore, preparation is an important prerequisite. Better still is a sensitive understanding by the drug user of the remitting and relapsing nature of heroin use. If this is understood by both drug user and therapist then success will be tempered by the awareness that relapse may occur and failure softened by the continued commitment to the treatment as an ongoing process.

Treatment Related to Individual Problems

Drug use may be heavy and damaging physically and psychologically for a period of months but is often followed by, or interspersed with, phases of comparatively light use or abstinence. Most heroin users, over a period of some years, will have long periods when either no drugs are taken or when non-dependent use is evident. In many individuals non-dependent use may be the predominant pattern of drug use and during this time physical and psychological well-being is apparent. Damaging or dependent drug use may be of short duration or absent completely. Evidence from the study of those surviving many years of heroin use is that, as time goes by, such non-dependent behaviour becomes more common and damaging behaviour less common. This 'maturing out' of drug use is discussed elsewhere in this book but is important in the context of treatment for obvious reasons. The on-off nature of all phases of heroin use is similarly vital to the present philosophy of management.

One must accept, therefore, that for reasons often outside the control of the therapist and even the patient, there will be good times and bad times, and that this will affect drug consumption. Treatment is more likely to be effective during a good phase and less effective during a bad one. It may sometimes be possible for anyone involved with a drug user to provoke the helpful situation or provide some of the requirements for a positive experience and, if this happens, then it will clearly aid therapy. Often, however, the therapist is in no position to know whether or not the time is right and so must proceed optimistically. The presence of several adverse factors may paradoxically provide the conditions required for improvement and most of those involved with drug users will have experienced the improvement consequent on situations which could get no worse.

During all stages of heroin use the possibility exists of spontaneous cure or abstinence. The first rule, as in all medical intervention, must be that we must do no harm. In a situation such as this, it might be difficult to see how the therapist could do any harm, but it is clear to many drug users that relapse or disappointment is commonly a result of injudicious medical intervention of an unsympathetic or even over-sympathetic nature. It might be argued that the provision of excessive supplies of alternative drugs may be a form of therapy which at best makes spontaneous remission less likely to happen and at worst is a source of a lethal supply of toxic drugs.

Implications of Controlled Drugtaking

If one accepts controlled drugtaking as being less damaging and therefore better, it is then possible for the first time to see an alternative approach to management and treatment as well as prevention of many problems. Without necessarily accepting that heroin use is a good or desirable thing, it is possible at least to intervene for the good of that individual and possibly for the good of society as a whole.

Controlled drugtaking implies an acceptance that it will be done regardless and therefore it is better done without harm. The problems, often unlike alcohol misuse, are usually related to confrontation with authority or damage from ill-informed drug use or poor and therefore dangerous administration. Intervention may therefore be to prevent some or all of these consequences over a period of time.

Without trying to ignore the obvious criticism of this type of intervention, such as the possibility of making problems worse by making drug use safer, it is important to consider first the positive possibilities. If one could eradicate the possibility of contamination and infection, this would undoubtedly reduce considerably the mortality and the illness problems which cost society so much. The potential for limiting the spread of AIDS and hepatitis B infection must be a major consideration. The damage done to society in material and spiritual forms by the alienation of drug misusers of all types is a reality only really understood by those close to the problem. Families of drug users suffer enormous agonies when a young adult suddenly adopts the appalling social stigma of the 'drug addict'. It is a staggering blow to them to recognize their family member as that outcast and only they can fully understand the injustice done by society. Somehow the damaging results of such attitudes should be altered to allow for the comparatively minor transgression of trying drugs on a casual basis. Without condoning drug use, it must be possible to recognize and offer support to those who have become involved rather than to cast out the offending individual.

Lack of Information Causing Failure of Treatment

Drug research has in some respects benefited from experiences related to alcohol problems. However, amidst the general ignorance there are some distinctive and important sources of research information about heroin users.

National studies in different countries indicate that large parts of the population use a variety of drugs, such as cannabis and amphetamines, and apparently come to no harm. Many of those who do come to the attention of doctors or other workers may recover spontaneously and probably do not go back to drug use. Of those who do get involved with 'damaging drug use' there is a significantly increased death rate, especially amongst those injecting heroin but also in those taking combinations of oral drugs.

Several prestigious studies have shown the periodicity of heroin use, that is, the on-off nature of drugtaking. This may lead to the conclusion, after studying the amount and frequency of drugtaking, that that individual is not dependent on the drug.

Waldorf and Winick have separately contributed much to the understanding of the changes that occur over a period of years in drug users, and Vaillant's long study of heroin in American users shows one third are not taking opiates and about half to be still using them in some form after seven years. All these studies, however, have been in groups of heroin users known to hospital clinics and therefore likely to be the worst examples of their type.

Thorley has pointed to what he calls the 'rush and trickle of abstinence' showing that a comparatively large number of heroin users stop in the first two or three years and that after that time there is a slow accumulation of additional abstainers resulting in totals of 40% or more after some ten years; the interest of this observation being the misleading final totals and the steadily decreasing abstaining rates over subsequent years. This, and much more, information is available and if it were collated, might lead to some conclusions about treatment without the need for further research. We know that some people die from using heroin, but not all, and not even a majority. Some continue to use opiates and some stop using them altogether. Some never become addicted, and some do but then apparently stop with no obvious treatment.

The big question must be whether or not these outcomes are influenced by therapy. The answer is not an easy one, primarily because changing social and medical policies have not allowed for adequate assessment of intervention. Stimson and Oppenheimer found 15% of heroin users to be dead at follow-up and stated that all died of drug-related causes. 38% were still receiving opiates from a drug dependence clinic. Thus during a ten year period of clinic availability in London the outcome was perhaps surprisingly good in simple terms of death and abstinence. It would be difficult to compare this evidence with the pre-1968 days when clinics were not available and much of the heroin, and other drugs in use in London, came from the overprescribing of a few doctors. Also the situation in the 1980s is somewhat different and therefore difficult to compare. Since the rapid escalation in numbers of young people using heroin, the clinics have rapidly been overwhelmed. Many researchers have observed that these agencies now see a group of heroin users, or ex-heroin users, in their early thirties who do not represent the new wave of problem drug users. Love and Gossop (1986) have observed that the vast increase in young individuals using heroin has lowered the average age recorded by the Home Office and that these people often have no contact with any agency, far less a drug dependence clinic.

Not only do we lack the information about treatment but we are now trying to treat a much larger group, a much younger group and probably a group with many other distinct differences. If the establishment of the clinic system in the UK did anything, then it cleaned up the problems left by inadequate control of prescribing in the 1960s. This has been recognized by many doctors and has been rejected as an adequate answer to the problem. Similar disenchantment with many methadone programmes in the US has arisen in both medical personnel and patients. The balance between control and treatment has in the 1970s been too much toward control and too little toward treatment. The initial moves towards treatment at the end of the 1970s with the establishment of drug treatment centres were followed by a lack of conviction about their role in the management of drug related problems. Thus, at the beginning of a new wave of heroin use, the existing centres were unable to respond in a meaningful way.

New Directions

Any new approach must take account of history and hopefully avoid the mistakes of the past. In addition it must offer something new or have some special relevance to a changed circumstance or an evolving problem.

Past experiences and mistakes have value in guiding future action. The problems of maintenance programmes and clinic management have been considerable, not the least being the institutionalization of individuals and the maintenance of their opiate dependence by the steady supply of substitute drugs. The 1970s therefore have established a cohort of opiate dependent individuals with little incentive to achieve abstinence and many reasons for not leaving the supply. The first half of the 1980s has seen a move towards tighter control, after the tendency to reduce this at the end of the 1970s. This however has taken a new and perhaps more sinister form. Decreasing resources but greater demands for health in the UK have prevented a move back to prescribing of maintenance therapy. Control has been the priority and the UK government strategy, published in March 1985, stressed the view that 'Stamping it (drug abuse) out will be slow and painful'. The plan includes:

1 Reducing supplies from abroad.
2 Tightening controls on drugs produced and prescribed here.
3 Making policing more effective.
4 Strengthening deterrents.
5 Improving prevention, treatment and rehabilitation.

Clearly the days of narrowly defining drug dependence as a disease are over. Only point 5 has any mention of treatment and rehabilitation and a further review of 'the strategy' reveals a minute financial commitment to these ends. A small allocation of money to a publicity campaign is now gone and will not be replaced and the government's own assessment of its effectiveness was substantial in its condemnation of this approach. The present British government clearly thinks the lesson it can learn from the past is that drug users have been treated too leniently and it is doing all it can to reverse this mistake.

Before analysing the past and suggesting pitfalls and mistakes to be avoided, one must consider any new factors which have come into the equation. What might influence the future approach to the heroin problem and how does it influence future policy changes? At a glance, the obvious newcomers to the field are the viruses responsible for hepatitis and AIDS. These may well change everything. They will undoubtedly influence potential newcomers to drug use and may prevent them ever starting. They may well account for many leaving the drug scene and they are bound to have some effect on drugtaking practices and behaviour. Finally, they are likely to account for a substantial increase in illness and death over the ensuing decade.

Both viruses are already endemic in the current heroin and cocaine injecting communities in most Western cities and the prevention opportunity has been lost. Yet again, society has shown its inability to predict and therefore prevent a new turn of events. It seems obvious now, but things usually do after they have happened.

Beside these problems other new features may seem unimportant, but there are several features of drug users of the 1980s that distinguish them from their predecessors and therefore point us to a different path for intervention. The spread of drug use away from the traditional centres (such as London and New York) and the declining age of onset of use indicate that the majority of heroin users have little or no contact with drug treatment centres, clinics or even experienced community workers. They may avoid detection and are likely to be distant from professional help during the critical first few months and years of their heroin using careers.

Future responses must understand the manifest failures of the past and should approach the present problem with a new pragmatism. The current situation is one of an enormous number of people infected or potentially infected (with the hepatitis and AIDS viruses), usually not living near a specialist unit and often not seeking help. If they have access to medical or appropriate educational information, it is through a non-specialist doctor or a local social or voluntary agency. None of these is equipped to offer complex or time-consuming therapy requiring supervision, prescription or special expertise. In view of the nature and location of the problem drugtakers of today, their problems must be dealt with in those communities and by those available. Thus, despite the recent British government report reaffirming the place of drug treatment in psychiatric institutions, the problem will present to non-specialists and therefore will be managed at that level. The failure of the Advisory Council in 1982 to recognize the extent and nature of the heroin problem of today has unfortunately left community services unprepared for this task and unsure of their role in coping with drug users. Are they part of the 'control' system as the clinics turned out to be, or are they offering genuine help and even treatment?

In the late 1980s therefore a similar situation exists to that in the late 1970s. An inadequate recognition of the problems of the 1960s led the Brain Committee to establish clinics to 'treat' the problems of drug use. The Advisory Council report at the beginning of the 1980s again responded inadequately to establish services and understanding of the problems now emerging.

9   New Directions

Observing the progression from the pre-control days when opiate use was not regarded as a problem, far less a disease, to the confusion and the increasing anxiety of the authorities in the fifties and sixties and the comparative calm of the seventies, one cannot help noticing how the problem has changed in nature throughout these times. At no time do the requirements for treatment and legislation seem to be the same as they were a few years previously. Nowhere is this more obvious than in the present decade, and never before has the legislation and availability of services been so apparently inadequate for the task in hand. The conflict between control of drugs and drugtakers and treatment has always been evident in one form or another and they have alternately taken precedence.

There would, however, seem to be a third force which is made up of both of these major factors and which exerts an invisible but vital influence. This is the views and attitudes of society towards the problem. If the mood of the public is towards control, then its influence will fall in line with the legal control authorities. If it is towards treatment, then it will pressurize allocation of resources and support for agencies supplying whatever treatment is in vogue. The power and influence of society to effect change is enormous and its responsibility correspondingly great.

Changing Attitudes

If attitudes were changing towards a more sympathetic understanding of the causes of heroin abuse, then AIDS has dealt this a severe blow. This new disease which has, in some areas, affected large numbers of heroin users has already reversed any softening of attitudes. The position of heroin users as a link by sexual contact with the wider society is likely to additionally decrease their popularity and increase the pressure to control heroin use by any means.

This is perhaps best seen at the present time by the moves in the United States to spend enormous sums of money on measures directly intended to control drugtakers and the availability of drugs. The House of Representatives recently considered proposals to use the armed forces to curb the flow of narcotics into that country, and to allow the use of illegally obtained evidence in drug trials. The increased use of illegal drugs is now seen as the biggest political issue at the present time. There are many reasons for these drastic invasions into areas previously regarded as inviolable civil liberties, and there will probably be pressure to invoke similar measures in other countries as the AIDS virus spreads. This failure of control will be seen as lack of resources or the lack of severity in dealing with drug users and drugtakers. Massachusetts Democrat, Brian Donnelly, was recently quoted in the New York Times as saying, 'I sure wouldn't want to be a drug pusher in this country when this (the anti drug bill) passes'.

Unfortunately, as has been observed in the past, this is unlikely to just apply to the 'pusher'. The average heroin user is about to feel the increasing wrath of a society which believes that failure in the past has been due to softness.

The slow erosion of our general misunderstanding of drugs and their effect is unlikely to stem such a tide of political and public concern and pressure. This is a change for the worse which looks set to happen and, although it may have a real effect in preventing some drug abuse, it may paradoxically make things worse in many areas. A particular aspect which will probably increase in severity is that of AIDS virus infections. In a climate of hostility, where punishment is severe, then communications between society and drug users become strained. Drugtakers become isolated and when they are contacted, are understandably suspicious and unlikely to accept information. Lines of communication with 'at risk' groups are vital in the control of this disease and the present situation has largely come about because of the alienation of those at risk. Society's lack of understanding of the risks they are taking and the rejection or estrangement of the drug users from sources of correct education have allowed the virus to spread.

Increasing the provision of funds to measures which seem to provide control over drug users is likely to allow rapid expansion of methadone programmes in the USA and to encourage the return of this type of treatment elsewhere.

The assumption that this type of therapy results in increased control is based on little substantial information. Moreover, the allocation of funds to this type of management will direct money and attention away from the more rational therapy discussed below. The perception that the problem is being dealt with will obscure the reality of drug use and AIDS virus spread in the community. Resources allocated to control AIDS virus spread rather than to treat or manage the problems giving rise to drug use are a futile attempt to treat an illness with an ineffective drug when the patient is already too ill to be saved.

The Likely Effect of AIDS

The expectation that AIDS will prevent young people using drugs through fear is something which cannot be taken for granted. It not only presupposes that they know about or understand the dangers, but fails to recognize the risk-taking inherent in adolescence and in drugtakers. Additionally it takes no account of the nature of AIDS as a disease and the presence in many countries of an established pool of infection amongst drug users and their contacts. New drugtakers may well be scared, but this disease is already present in most cities in Europe and North America, if not worldwide. There will still be those who use drugs despite the fear and those who use in ignorance. Sexual spread in drug users and non-drug users is likely to ensure the progress of AIDS in the future. Thus the present focus of infection in such groups as homosexual men and drug injectors may well change in the next few years. The early presence in these groups may well be purely because of the ability of the virus to spread rapidly amongst those people.

Risk Reduction

Accepting that drug abuse is endemic in many societies and that many measures have failed to eradicate or even to improve this situation, a sensible policy for the future is much needed. The causes of most of the physical damage related to heroin taking by injection has suddenly become all too clear. The AIDS virus has focused attention on the infective nature of many of the problems. Drug users infected with the AIDS virus might well ask why nobody warned them of this particular danger as soon as the disease was recognized as a bloodborne infection. Indeed, there are many drug users unaware of these dangers even now.

Table 9.1 (p. 118) shows a list of problems directly related to heroin abuse or present in those in direct contact with an infected individual.

Although this is incomplete, there seem to be areas in which education or intervention might prevent damaging results. An obvious feature is the preponderance of infectious agents causing problems. This is not to say that the problems lower down the list are less severe, but only that infection lends itself to prevention more easily than social problems or financial predicaments, which tend to be unique to each individual situation.

An example of a potentially preventable epidemic of infection in drug injectors is demonstrated by what happened in Edinburgh during 1983 and 1984. Figure 9.1 (p. 119) shows a rapid rise in the numbers of individuals infected with the AIDS virus in a short period of time. A similar graph could be drawn for the hepatitis B infection, which spreads in the same way by the use of infected needles and syringes.

Table 9.1   *Preventable problems*

HIV exposure by needle sharing
HIV exposure by sexual contact
Pregnancy in HIV infected female
Pregnancy in potentially infected female
Pregnancy in hepatitis B carrier female
Hepatitis B exposure by needle sharing
Hepatitis B exposure by sexual contact
Fungal infection of eyes (endophthalmitis)
Heart valve infection (endocarditis)
Injection site problem (infected)
Injection site problem (non-infected)
Thrombosis (clots in veins)
Thrombosis (clots in arteries)
Fatal overdosage of one drug
Fatal overdosage of combination of drugs
Non-fatal overdosage of drug or drugs
Amenorrhoea
Weight loss
Malnutrition
Other drug abuse – illegal
                 – legal
                 – cigarettes
                 – alcohol
                 – prescribed
Emotional problems
Social problems
Family problems
Financial problems

Risk reduction therefore is largely about recognizing problems as they arise or even before they arise. The supply of appropriate information, education or intervention directed at a particular problem might be expected to be more specific than just a blanket message for all drug users. The fact that cure is unlikely in the short term has to be accepted and help offered on a different basis. The personal problems in an individual at any one time should be recognized and addressed.

Understanding that heroin users are subject to normal, or even excessive, pressures present in the life of any person allows for help to be offered for those problems which may be preventing the cessation of drug use.

Local Problems – Local Solutions

The move toward community management of drug problems has been a positive development in many ways. It has allowed for local concentration on problems predominant in that area.

It is well known that drug misuse has many patterns and what may be an appropriate facility in one area may be totally useless in another. Special expertise is always necessary but it is only useful when coupled with local knowledge and awareness of behaviour in that area. Traditionally poor communications between drug using communities and professionals have meant that problems can arise without warning and in an advanced state. Thus the first knowledge of infection in a group of drug users may be when they arrive in hospital suffering from or dying of a specific disease.

The concentration on risk reduction measures such as the supply of advice about sterile injection technique is only of use in an area where people inject drugs in a dangerous way. In an area where heroin is inhaled, it may easily make a situation worse if needles and syringes are supplied legally. Similarly intense education about heroin use is seen by many as potentially damaging if

Fig. 9.1 *Cumulative number of first positive HIV antibody test results amongst 83 IVDAs by year quarters*

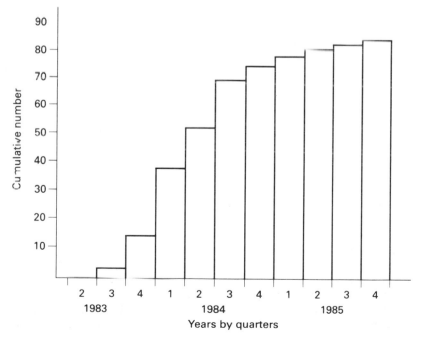

directed at groups who previously had little interest or information about drugs.

In the same way, types of drugs taken vary from place to place and the current interest in one city may be quite distinct from another. Information about heroin abuse may be quite redundant in a city where amphetamines are widely used or amongst a group predominantly taking cocaine.

Specific local problems require individual solutions and specific local information is the important requirement before solutions can be considered.

Implicit in any policy of risk reduction is the prevention of infection through the injection of contaminated materials. In common with many aspects of control of drug misuse, the control of sterile equipment is incomplete. Retrospectively, it is rather difficult to see any pattern or logic in the control of syringe and needle availability. Since the invention of the hypodermic needle and syringe in 1853, control of its use has been sporadic and variable. In modern times patterns of control have emerged where there was a perceived need for it and have been non-existent elsewhere. At the present time there are very few States in the US where there is legislation on needle and syringe availability. Significantly these States account for the monopoly of drug abuse.

In Europe attitudes vary from the extreme of the Netherlands, where needles and syringes are available on a return basis at a nominal charge with a higher cost when no old equipment is brought back, to the puritan prohibition in Scotland. The regional variation in the UK has emerged from the failure of national policy to implement uniform practice and the provision of 13,000 clean needles over the counter in London during 1984 (Evans 1985) makes a stark contrast to other areas of the country. Such provision of sterile equipment is unlikely to solve all the problems associated with heroin use, but without it the problems of AIDS will get more severe.

Risk reduction or damage limitation is not meant to be a panacea or a measure to be taken in isolation from other ways of preventing and dealing with drug misuse. It is purely a way of avoiding or preventing some of the major dangers and tragedies in individual patients and amongst groups of drug users. Used in this way, it may help to stop problems of damaging behaviour or provide the necessary support or incentive to drug users to help themselves.

In the same way as the design of a safer car or the use of a seat belt might be expected to limit the dangers of driving a car, risk reduction measures may reduce or prevent damage in certain situations.

Contacting Drug Misusers

One of the greatest problems encountered by those involved with drugtakers is the lack of suitable opportunities for providing appropriate medical and educational material. Although the typical 'junkie' may come in contact repeatedly with many services, the larger group of controlled or experimenting users does not. The size of this group is unknown although Nightingale (1977) in the US estimated that, while there are approximately 150,000 to 170,000 getting some form of treatment and another 100,000 in gaol for drug related offences at any one time, there are another 300,000 to 400,000 who have never sought professional help for drug problems.

The usual criteria used to detect opiate users, acquisition of infectious disease, arrest rates, overdose deaths, treatment programme attendance, are all designed to confirm the stereotype of uncontrolled drug users. Such data seem only to reinforce this extreme view of heroin use.

Many of the failures in drug misuse therapy may be related to this difficulty in contacting those who might benefit most from help. A national study by Abelson and Fishburne in 1976 in the US showed that 1.2% of adults had had experience with heroin and in the same year Hunt and Chambers estimated that there were three to four million heroin users in that country. They added, however, that probably only 10% were dependent on the drug. Thus a majority of heroin users have no direct contact with agencies designed to treat or help.

Research

There have been many substantial contributions to the literature relating to the use and misuse of drugs. When related to heroin, cocaine and cannabis, most contributions have been largely descriptive and confined to small areas of interest. Thus the obsession with treating withdrawal symptoms and the behaviour of patients attending methadone maintenance clinics have revealed much information about these aspects of opiate-related behaviour, but have prevented the close examination of abstinence which occurs without any treatment. In an effort to show how people can be weaned off heroin, it has not been demonstrated that, at least in some individuals, this occurs spontaneously without any treatment. Zinberg (1979) has drawn attention to the many inconsistencies in the 'addictive' view of opiate use and opened up vast new areas of research possibilities with vital implications for how opiate users may be helped either in the clinic or in society.

The concentration of research in academic institutions and in hospital centres has consistently selected those individuals who are worst affected, who cope with drug abuse least well or who merely cope with it in a form easily recognizable to the physicians. Those attending maintenance programmes over a period of years may long since have ceased to demonstrate anything other than institutionalized opiate dependent behaviour. What is worse is that these rather narrow research focuses continue to reinforce a set of values and characteristics about heroin, or other drug use, which do not reflect what may happen outside an institution or in the lives of those not forced into the mould of the disturbed and severely dependent individual.

Society's views represent what information it has on a topic. Thus the grossly misleading information on the use and safety of cannabis in the 1960s was believed by a large percentage of the population. Current views, based on more precise information, are able to objectively assess a drug and its dangers. As a result a new era of awareness has a more reasoned perspective and allows for a diminution in anxiety and misunderstanding.

More precise understanding of the relationship between drugtaking and such factors as unemployment, social deprivation, lack of opportunities and environmental conditions may give rise to a new view of heroin. Research into the damaging effects of a drug like heroin can only be carried out effectively if those involved ask the right questions and are prepared to accept the answers. If the answers suggest that heroin use is self-limiting and that the dangers are largely due to ignorance, violence, infection and an expression of distrust in an individual, then these are the problems to be tackled. Good research should result in a change in something, whether that be attitudes or the practice of those involved. Continued research reveals that patterns are constantly changing in all countries. Robins observed that while non-dependent drug use was infrequent in the period 1930–1950, such use had become widespread by 1976. Her review of the progress of American personnel who had served in Vietnam (1976) observed continual heroin use in about 20% of individuals known to have used while in S.E. Asia.

Heroin use, like the societies in which it exists, will change but is unlikely to go away.

Perspective

A new perception of heroin from the perspective of our knowledge of non-dependent use, controlled use and risk reduction allows the physician or other professional to intervene in a non-confrontational way. No longer is he trying to cure this person of an evil influence or disease. Moreover, the confusion over prescribing should be seen as serving only to prevent dialogue or progression. The real issues of preventing damage and passing on information should be allowed to take precedence.

Removing the tension and changing attitudes from punitive to palliative is the first vital step in helping drug users. Increasingly, accurate information about the nature of heroin abuse and those who use the drug but never appear to suffer the damaging consequences is urgently required, partly to shed some light on difficult areas of understanding behaviour but principally to defuse the damaging idea of heroin use as a major threat to society.

A prohibitionist public policy based on superficial analysis of those chaotic users and with the underlying assumption that all heroin use leads to dependency has led us to a pitch of confusion. What is the damage being done and to whom? If it exists, is the crisis for society, for families of drug users or for drug users themselves? The elusive nature of the drugs problem may well cause panic and major ripples through all sectors of society, but so would many other issues presented in the same way.

Much of the international anxiety about heroin abuse is created by the way it is presented. Many other more devastating problems exist which, given similar exposure, would cause a corresponding reaction. Legal drug use, deaths from road traffic accidents, violence and trauma all present much more alarming death rates and damage to society. Potential pandemics such as nuclear war, famine or natural disasters will touch much more of the world's population than heroin ever will. If the damage seen to be caused by heroin were attributed to the reason the individual gave for starting the drug, then the real problems might begin to be apparent.

That heroin use is dangerous and that dependence may sometimes exist is not in dispute, but if young people are continually faced with choices about drugs, then the real risks, the real dangers and the real solutions are the ones we urgently need to understand.

Research of the changing nature of drug use and drug users can only be done in the community and will only be of value if it is gathered in combination with a sympathetic understanding of problems and individuals. High technology has little to offer drug users and the preoccupation of society with solutions provided by this type of research is part of the problem.

A recent New England study (McAuliffe *et al.* 1986) revealed that 59% of physicians and 78% of the students questioned had used psychoactive drugs at one time or another. 10% of the physicians reported current regular drug use (once a month or more often). The drugs involved were most commonly cocaine, cannabis and heroin. Drug use is not the preserve of the insane or the eccentric fringe and educated people are clearly making choices in their lives which involve a variety of drugs. If the dangers are real then correct information must be made available and if increasingly sophisticated drugtakers are to be educated then the time to do it is before they arrive in a hospital unit.

References

ABELSON, H. I. and FISHBURNE, P. M. (1976) *Non medical use of psychoactive substances: 1975/1976 Nationwide Study among Youth and Adults, Princeton, NJ*. Response Analysis Corporation.

ADVISORY COUNCIL ON THE MISUSE OF DRUGS. (1984) *Prevention*. Home Office, London.

ALEXANDER, M. (1974) Surveillance of heroin related deaths in Atlanta 1971–1973. *JAMA*, 229: 677–678.

ALTER, A. A. and MICHAEL, M. (1958) Serum hepatitis in a group of drug addicts. *New England Journal of Medicine*, 259: 387.

ALTMAN, D. (1986) *AIDS and the New Puritanism*. Pluto, London.

ASHTON, H. (1984) Benzodiazepine withdrawal: an unfinished story. *British Medical Journal*, 288: 1135–40.

BANKS, A. and WALLER, T. A. N. (1983) *Drug Addiction and Polydrug Abuse*. ISDD, London.

BERRIDGE, V. and EDWARDS, G. (1981) *Opium and the People*. Allan Lane, London.

BEWLEY, T. H., BEN-ARIE, O., JAMES, I. P. (1968) Morbidity and mortality from heroin dependence. 1. Survey of heroin addicts known to the Home Office. *British Medical Journal*, 1: 725–726.

BEWLEY, T. H., GHODSE, A. H. (1983) Unacceptable face of private practice: prescription of controlled drugs to addicts. *British Medical Journal*, 286: 1876–1877.

BLACK, D. (1986) *The Plague Years: A Chronicle of AIDS, the Epidemic of Our Time*. Picador, London.

BOWMAN, W. C. and RAND, M. J. (1980) *Textbook of pharmacology*. 2nd ed. Blackwell Scientific Publications, Oxford.

BRATTER, T. E. (1974) The crime of methadone maintenance treatment programs: A conspiracy against the heroin addict, In: MILLER, L. (ed.) *Abstracts of the Third International Symposium on Drug Abuse, Jerusalem, Israel*. Graphress Ltd, 58–59.

BUCKNALL, A. B. V. and ROBERTSON, J. R. (1985) Heroin misuse and family medicine. *Family Practice*, 2, 4: 244–251.

BUCKNALL, A. B. V. and ROBERTSON, J. R. (1986) Deaths of heroin users in a general practice population 1986. *Journal of the Royal College of General Practitioners*, 36: 120–122.

BUCKNALL, A. B. V., ROBERTSON, J. R. and STRACHAN, T. G. (1986) Use of psychiatric drug treatment services by heroin users from general practice. *British Medical Journal*, 292: 997–999.

BURR, A. (1984) The illicit non-pharmaceutical heroin market and drug scene in Kensington Market. *British Journal of Addiction*, 79, 337–344.

BURROUGHS, W. (1957) *Junkie*. New English Library, London.

BURROUGHS, W. (1959) *The Naked Lunch*. Corgi Books, London.

CONNELL, P. H. (1958) *Amphetamine Psychosis*. Oxford University Press, London.

COTTRELL, D., CHILDS-CLARK, A., GHODSE, A. H. (1985) British opiate addicts: an eleven year follow-up. *British Journal of Psychiatry*, 146: 448–450.

DEL ORTO, A. (1974) The role and resources of the family during the rehabilitation process. *Journal of Psychadelic Drugs*, 6: 435–445.

DEPARTMENT OF HEALTH AND SOCIAL SECURITY (1982) Treatment and rehabilitation: report of the advisory council on the misuse of drugs. HMSO, London.

DEPARTMENT OF HEALTH AND SOCIAL SECURITY (1984) *Guidelines of Good Clinical Practice in the Treatment of Drug Misuse*. HMSO, London.

DITTON, J. and SPEIRITS, K. (1981) The rapid increase in heroin addiction in Glasgow during 1981. Background paper No. 2. Department of Sociology, University of Glasgow.

DOLE, V. P. and NYSWANDER, M. E. (1967) A medical treatment for diacetylmorphine (heroin) addiction – a clinical trial with methadone hydrochloride. *JAMA*, 193: 646–650.

DORN, N. and SOUTH, N. (1985) *Helping Drug Users*. Gower, London.

DUMONT, M. P. (1973) The junkie as political enemy. *American Journal on Ortho-psychiatry*, 43, 4: 537–539.

EDWARDS, G. and BUSCH, C. (eds) (1981) *Drug Problems in Britain – A Review of Ten Years*. Academic Press, London.

EVANS, C. (1985) Information pack 3 for Drug Advisory Committee. Directorate of Social Services, London Borough of Tower Hamlets.

FAZEY, C. (1977) *The Aetiology of Psychoactive Substance use*. UNESCO, Paris.

FIELD, T. (1985) *Escaping the Dragon*. Unwin, London.

FOLLETT, E. A. C., MCINTYRE, A., O'DONNELL, B., CLEMENTS, G. B., DESSELBERGER, U. (1986) HTLV 3 antibody in drug abusers in the west of Scotland: the Edinburgh connection. *Lancet*, i: 446–447.

FUCHS, D., DIERICH, M. P., HAUSEN, A. *et al.* (1985) Are homosexuals less at risk of AIDS than intravenous drug abusers and haemophiliacs? *Lancet*, ii: 1130.

GHODSE, A. H., SHEENAN, M., TAYLOR, C. and EDWARDS, G. (1985) Deaths of drug addicts in the UK 1967–1981. *British Medical Journal*, 290: 425–428.

GOODMAN, L. S. (1985) *The Pharmacological Basis of Therapeutics*. Collier Macmillan, West Drayton.

GOSSOP, M. (1982) *Living with Drugs*. Temple Smith, London.

HANCOCK, G. and CARIM, E. (1986) *A.I.D.S. The Deadly Epidemic*. Victor Gollancz Ltd, London.

HARTNOLL, R., DAVIAND, I., LEWIS, R. and MITCHESON, M. (1985) *Drug Problems: Assessing Local Needs (A practical manual for assessing the nature and extent of problematic drug use in a community)*. Drug Indicators Project, London.

HAVE TEN, H., SPORKEN, P. (1985) Heroin addiction, ethics and philosophy of medicine. *Journal of Medical Ethics*, 11: 173–177.

HAW, S. (1985) *Drug Problems in Greater Glasgow*. Chameleon Press, London.

HEATHER, N. (ed.) (1985) *The Misuse of Alcohol*. Croom Helm, London.

HEATHER, N. and ROBERTSON, I. (1981) *Controlled Drinking*. Methven, London.

HENSMAN, C. and ZACUNE, J. (1971) *Drugs, Alcohol and Tobacco in Britain*. Heinemann Ltd, London.

HOME OFFICE (1984) Statistics of the misuse of drugs in the United Kingdom (1983). *Home Office Statistics Bulletin*, London.

HOME OFFICE (1985) *Tackling Drug Misuse: A Summary of the Government's Strategy*. HMSO, London.

HOME OFFICE (1985) Statistics on the Misuse of Drugs in the United Kingdom (1984). *Home Office Statistics Bulletin*, London.

HOUSE OF COMMONS (1985) Social Services Committee on the Misuse of Drugs.

HUNT, D. G. and CHAMBERS, C. D. (1976) *The Heroin Epidemics: A Study of Heroin Use in the United States 1965–1975*. Spectrum, New York.

JENINEK, E. M. (1960) *The Disease Concept of Alcoholism*. Millhouse Press, New Haven.

JOE, G. W., LEISHMAN, D. N. *et al.* (1982) Addict death rates during a four-year post-treatment follow-up. *American Journal of Public Health*, 72: 703–709.

KAPLAN, J. (1983) *The Hardest Drug – Heroin and Public Policy*, University of Chicago Press, Chicago.

KAUFMAN, E., KAUFMAN, P. N. (eds) (1979) *Family Therapy of Drug and Alcohol Abuse*. Gardner Press, New York.

KLATZMAN, D., GLUCKMAN, J. C. (1986) HIV infection: facts and hypotheses. *Immunology Today*, 7(10): 291–295.

KOSTEN, T. R. and KLEBER, H. D. (1984) Strategies to improve compliance with narcotic antagonists. *American Journal of Drug and Alcohol Abuse*, 10: 249.

LAZZARIN, A., GALLI, M., GEROLDI, D., ZANETTI, A., CROCCHIOCO, P., AIUTI, F., MORONI, M. (1985) Epidemic of HTLV 3/LAV infection in drug addicts in Milan: Serological survey and clinical follow-up. *Infection* 13(5): 216–218.

LOURIA, D. B. (1970) *The Drug Scene*. Corgi Books, London.

LOVE, J., and GOSSOP, M. (1985) The process of referral and disposal within a London drug dependency clinic. *British Journal of Addiction*, 80: 435–440.

MCAULIFFE, W. E., ROTHMAN, M. *et al.* (1986) Psychoactive drug use among practising physicians and medical students. *New England Journal of Medicine*, 315: 805–810.

MAISTO, S. A., SOBELL, L. C., SOBELL, M. B. (1982) Corroboration of drug abusers' self reports through the use of multiple data sources. *American Journal of Drug and Alcohol Abuse*, 9(3): 301–308.

MARLATT, G. A., GEORGE, W. H. (1984) Relapse prevention and overview of the model. *British Journal of Addiction*, 79: 261–273.

MARMOR, M., DES JARLAIS, D. C., FRIEDMAN, S. R., LYNDEN, M., EL-SADR, W. (1984) The epidemic of acquired immunodeficiency syndrome (AIDS) and suggestions for its control in drug abusers. *Journal of Substance Abuse and Treatment*, 1: 237–247.

MARTIN, W. R., JASINSKI, D. R., MANSKY, P. A. (1973) Naltrexone, an antagonist for the treatment of heroin dependence. *Archives of General Psychiatry*, 28: 784–791.

MELBYE, M. (1986) The natural history of human T lymphotropic virus III infection: the cause of AIDS. *British Medical Journal*, 292: 5–12.

MILLER, D., WEBER, J. and GREEN, J. (eds) (1986) *The Management of A.I.D.S. Patients*. Macmillan, London.

NATIONAL COMMISSION ON MARIJUANA AND DRUG ABUSE (1972) *Drug Use in America: Problems in Perspective.* US Government Printing Department, Washington DC.

NEWMAN, R. G. (1985) The need to redefine 'addiction'. *New England Journal of Medicine*, 308: 1096–1098.

NIGHTINGALE, S. (1977) Treatment for drug abusers in the United States. *Addict Dis*, 3: 11–20.

PANOS INSTITUTE (1986) Aids and the Third World. The Panos Institute, Panos Dossier 1, London.

PAULUS, I. (1966) *A Comparative Study of Long-term and Short-term Withdrawal of Narcotic Addicts Voluntarily Seeking Comprehensive Treatment.* Narcotic Addiction Foundation of British Columbia, Vancouver, Canada.

PHILLIPSON, R. V. (1970) *Modern Trends In Drug Dependence and Alcoholism.* Butterworths, London.

PINCHING, A. J., JEFFRIES, D. J. (1985) AIDS and the HTLV 3/LAV infection: consequences for obstetrics and prenatal medicine. *British Journal of Obstetrics and Gynaecology*, 92: 1211–1217.

PLANT, M. A. (1981) What Aetiologies? In: EDWARDS, G. and BUSCH, C. (eds) *Drug Problems in Britain: A Review of Ten Years.* Academic Press, London.

PLANT, M. A. (1985) *Women, Drinking and Pregnancy.* Tavistock, London.

PLANT, M. A., PECK, D. F. and SAMUEL, E. (1985) *Alcohol, Drugs and School-leavers.* Tavistock, London.

PLANT, M. L. (ed.) (1982) *Drinking and Problem Drinking.* Junction Books, London.

ROBERTSON, J. R., BUCKNALL, A. B. V. (1986) Abstinence, controlled and dependent use of heroin: drug takers with minimal intervention. Report of Edinburgh Drug Addiction Society: SHHD.

ROBERTSON, J. R., BUCKNALL, A. B. V. and WIGGINS, P. (1986) Regional variations in H.I.V. antibody seropositivity in British intravenous drug users. *Lancet*, i: 1435–36.

ROBERTSON, J. R., BUCKNALL, A. B. V., WELSBY, P. D., ROBERTS, J. J. K., INGLIS, J. M., PEUTHERER, J. F., BRETTLE, R. P. (1986) Epidemic of A.I.D.S. related virus (HTLV3/LAV) infection among intravenous drug users. *British Medical Journal*, 292: 527–529.

ROBINS, L. N. and MURPHY, G. E. (1967) Drug use in a normal population of young negro men. *American Journal of Public Health*, 570: 1580–1596.

ROBINS, L. N., HELZER, J. E. and DAVIS, D. M. (1976) Narcotic use in S.E. Asia and afterwards: an interview study of 898 Vietnam returnees. *Arch Gen Psych*, 32: 955–61.

ROLLESTON COMMITTEE (1926) Report of the Departmental Committee on Morphine and Heroin Addiction. HMSO, London.

ROSENHAM, D. L. (1973) On being sane in insane places. *Science*, 179: 250–258.

ROUNSAVILLE, B. J., WEISMANN, M. M., WILBER, C. H., KLEBER, H. D. (1982) Pathways to opium addiction: an evaluation of differing antecedents. *British Journal of Psychiatry*, 141: 437–446.

ROYAL COLLEGE OF PHYSICIANS (1983) *Health or Smoking?* Pitman, London.

ROYAL COLLEGE OF PSYCHIATRISTS (1986) *Alcohol: Our Favourite Drug.* Tavistock, London.

RUTTENBER, A. J., LUKE, J. L. (1974) Heroin related deaths: new epidemiological insights. *Science*, 226: 14–20.

SACKMAN, B. S., SACKMAN, M. M., DE ANGELIS, G. G. (1978) Heroin addiction as an occupation: traditional addicts and heroin addicted polydrug abusers. *International Journal of Addiction*, 13: 427–441.

SCHOENBAUM, E. E., SELWYN, P. A., KLEIN, R. S. *et al.* (1986) Prevalence of and risk factors associated with HTLV3/LAV antibodies among intravenous drug users in Methadone Program in New York City. (Communication 198: 534b) Paris AIDS Conference, June.

SIEGEL, S., HINSON, R. E. KRANK, M. D., MCCULLY, J. (1982) Heroin 'overdose' deaths: contribution of drug-associated environmental users. *Science*, 216: 436–437.

SPIRA, T. J., DES JARLAIS, D. C., MARMOR, M. *et al.* (1984) Prevalence of antibody to lymphodenopathy associated virus among drug-detoxification patients in New York. *New England Journal of Medicine*, 331: 467–468.

STEINBERG, N. (ed.) (1969) *Scientific Basis of Drug Dependence*. Churchill Ltd, London.

STIMSON, G. V. and OPPENHEIMER, E. (1982) *Heroin Addiction Treatment and Control in Britain*. Tavistock, London.

SUSMAN, J. (ed.) (1972) *Drug Use and Social Policy*. AMS Press, New York.

THORLEY, A. (1981) Longitudinal studies of drug dependence. In: EDWARDS, G. and BUSCH, C. (eds) *Drug Problems in Britain*. Academic Press, London.

TREBACH, A. S. (1982) *The Heroin Solution*. Yale University Press, New Haven.

VAILLANT, G. E. (1966) A twelve year follow-up of New York narcotic addicts: 1. The relation of treatment to outcome. *American Journal of Psychiatry*, 122: 727–37.

VAILLANT, G. E. (1973) A twenty year follow-up of New York narcotic addicts. *Archives of General Psychiatry*, 29, 237–241.

WALDORF, D. (1972) Life without heroin: some social adjustment during long term periods of voluntary abstention. In: SUSMAN, J. (ed.) *Drug Use and Social Policy*. AMS Press, New York.

WILLE, R. (1981) Ten year follow-up of a representative sample of London heroin addicts; clinic attendance, abstinence and mortality. *British Journal of Addiction*, 76: 259–266.

WILLE, R. (1983) Process of recovery from heroin dependence: relationship to treatment, social change and drug use. *Journal of Drug Issues*, 13: 333–342.

WILLIAMS, J. B. (ed.) (1967) *Narcotics and Hallucinogens – A Handbook*. Glencoe Press, California.

WINICK, C. (1962) Maturing out of narcotic addiction. *Bulletin of Narcotics*, 14: 1–7.

WORLD HEALTH ORGANIZATION (1977) *International Classification of Diseases*. WHO, Geneva.

ZELSON, C., RUBIO, E., WASSERMAN, E. (1971) Neonatal narcotic addiction ten year observation. *Paediatius*, 48: 178–189.

ZINBERG, N. E. (1979) Non addictive opiate user. In: DUPONT, R. L., GOLDSTEIN, A. and O'DONNEL, J. (eds) *Handbook on Drug Abuse*. NIDA, Rockville.

ZINBERG, N. E. (1984) *Drug, Set and Setting*. Yale University Press, New Haven.

Index